Notes on Medical Virology

CHURCHILL LIVINGSTONE MEDICAL TEXTS

Notes on Infectious Diseases
A.P. Ball

Epidemiology in Medical Practice
Second edition
D.J.P. Barker and G. Rose

Pain: Its Nature, Analysis and Treatment
Michael R. Bond

Essentials of Dermatology
J.L. Burton

Essential Ophthalmology
H. Chawla

Notes on Psychiatry
Fifth edition
I.M. Ingram, G.C. Timbury and R.M. Mowbray

Physiology: A Clinical Approach
Third edition
G.R. Kelman

A Concise Textbook of Gastroenterology
Second edition
M.J.S. Langman

Tumours: Basic Principles and Clinical Aspects
Christopher Louis

Nutrition and its Disorders
Third edition
Donald S. McLaren

The Essentials of Neuroanatomy
Third edition
G.A.G. Mitchell and D. Mayor

An Introduction to Primary Medical Care
Second edition
David Morrell

Urology and Renal Medicine
Third edition
J.E. Newsam and J.J.B. Petrie

Clinical Bacteriology
P.W. Ross

Sexually Transmitted Diseases
Third edition
C.B.S. Schofield

Notes on Medical Bacteriology
J.D. Sleigh and Morag C. Timbury

An Introduction to General Pathology
Second edition
W.G. Spector

Child Psychiatry for Students
Second edition
Frederick H. Stone and Cyrille Koupernik

Introduction to Clinical Endocrinology
Second edition
John A. Thomson

Clinical Pharmacology
Third edition
P. Turner and A. Richens

Immunology: An Outline for Students of Medicine and Biology
Fourth edition
D.M. Weir

Clinical Thinking and Practice: Diagnosis and Decision in Patient Care
H.J. Wright and D.B. MacAdam

LIVINGSTONE MEDICAL TEXTS

Geriatric Medicine for Students
J.C. Brocklehurst and T. Hanley

An Introduction to Clinical Rheumatology
William Carson Dick

Introduction to Clinical Examination
Second edition
Edited by John Macleod

Psychological Medicine for Students
John Pollitt

Respiratory Medicine
Malcolm Schonell

Cardiology for Students
Max Zoob

Notes on Medical Virology

Morag C. Timbury
M.D., Ph.D., F.R.S.E., F.R.C.P (Glasg.), F.R.C. Path.
Titular Professor and William Teacher Lecturer,
University of Glasgow, Department of Bacteriology,
Royal Infirmary, Glasgow

FOREWORD BY
J.H. Subak-Sharpe
B.Sc., Ph.D., F.R.S.E.
Professor of Virology, University of Glasgow

SEVENTH EDITION

CHURCHILL LIVINGSTONE
EDINBURGH LONDON MELBOURNE AND NEW YORK 1983

CHURCHILL LIVINGSTONE
Medical Division of Longman Group Limited

Distributed in the United States of America by
Churchill Livingstone Inc., 1560 Broadway, New
York, N.Y. 10036, and by associated companies,
branches and representatives throughout the world.

First edition 1967
Second edition 1969
Third edition 1971
Fourth edition 1973
Fifth edition 1974
Sixth edition 1978
ELBS edition first published 1978
Seventh edition 1983
    Reprinted 1984

ISBN 0 443 02699 8

British Library Cataloguing in Publication Data
Timbury, Morag C.
    Notes on medical virology. — 7th ed. — (Churchill
    Livingstone medical texts)
    1. Viruses   2. Micro-organisms, Pathogenic
    I. Title
    616'.0194   QR360

Library of Congress Cataloging in Publication Data
Timbury, Morag Crichton.
    Notes on medical virology.

    (Churchill Livingstone medical text)
    Bibliography: p.
    Includes index.
    1. Virus diseases.   I. Title.   II. Series.
    RC114.5.T55   1982   616'.0194   82-1140
                                          AACR2

Printed in Singapore by Selector Printing Co Pte Ltd

Foreword

Virology concerns itself with viruses at many different levels — from the study at the molecular level of the structure, genetic information, content and function of the particle and the virus-host cell complex, via the analysis of the events which define the progress of viral disease in the host organism to interrelationships between the virus and populations of potential host organisms. These different levels necessarily have led to a dichotomy of virology into the pure and the applied field and, until now, medicine for all practical purposes has been almost solely concerned with the latter. But, as our knowledge of viruses at all analytical levels is becoming more and more extensive, and particularly if one considers the recent dramatic increase of our understanding of events at the molecular level, some knowledge of the general field of pure virology is bound to become relevant even for the doctor in general practice whose sole concern in the past has been with the field of applied virology. These notes are starting to bridge this gap.

Dr Timbury's lucid, concise and astonishingly comprehensive book of notes is particularly well suited to help medical students, who are primarily concerned with the spectrum of diseases caused by viruses, to get acquainted with the subject of virology. The book neither aims nor pretends to be a self-sufficient textbook, and, to this end, recommended books for further reading have been included. Clearly presented, informative and inexpensive, this book should prove most useful to students in conjunction with their course of lectures, practicals and hospital instruction.

The book, which is an excellent summary of the major virological problems in medicine, can be highly recommended for students of medicine.

J.H. Subak-Sharpe

Preface

This book originated from lecture notes which were handed out to accompany my virology lectures to the medical students in Glasgow University. I wrote it in the same concise note form to try and present clearly the facts about virus diseases which students have to know for their professional examination in microbiology. Although it is meant to be reasonably comprehensive, students should refer to some of the larger books on the subject and I have listed some of my favourites on page 147.

Many colleagues have helped me with advice and discussion on numerous points, notably Professors C.R. Madeley and T.H. Pennington and Doctors Eleanor J. Bell, E.A.C. Follett, Joan Macnab, C.R. Pringle and R.G. Sommerville. Thanks are also due to Dr Follett, Dr Helen Laird and Professor Madeley for the photographs and to Mr R. Callander for the drawings and diagrams.

Finally I should like to thank Professor J.H. Subak-Sharpe, not only for the Foreword but for the many happy years I spent in his department, and Professor N.R. Grist in whose laboratory I first acquired my interest in viruses.

Glasgow 1983   Morag C. Timbury

Contents

1

General properties of viruses

Viruses are the smallest known infective agents. Most forms of life — animals, plants and bacteria — are susceptible to infection with appropriate viruses.

Three main properties distinguish viruses from other micro-organisms:

1. *Small size.* Viruses are smaller than other organisms and vary in size from 10 nm to 300 nm. In contrast, bacteria are approximately 1000 nm and erythrocytes are 7500 nm in diameter.
2. *Genome.* The genome of viruses may be either DNA or RNA; viruses contain only one type of nucleic acid.
3. *Metabolically inert.* Viruses have no metabolic activity outside susceptible host cells; they do not possess any ribosomes or protein-synthesising apparatus although some viruses contain enzymes within their particles; viruses cannot therefore multiply in inanimate media but only inside living cells. On entry into a susceptible cell, however, the virus genome or nucleic acid is transcribed into — or itself acts as — virus-specific messenger RNA which then directs the replication of new virus particles.

STRUCTURE OF VIRUSES

Viruses consist basically of a core of nucleic acid surrounded by a protein coat.

The protein coat is antigenic and specific for each virus type; it protects the viral genome from inactivation by adverse environmental factors, e.g. nucleases in the blood stream.

The structures which make up a virus particle are known as:

Virion — the intact virus particle.

Capsid — the protein coat.

Capsomeres — the protein structural units of which the capsid is composed.

Nucleic acid.

Envelope: the particles of many viruses are surrounded by a lipo-protein envelope containing viral antigens but also partially derived from the outer membrane of the host cell.

Virus particles show three types of symmetry:

Cubic — in which the particles are icosahedral protein shells with the nucleic acid contained inside (Fig. 1.1).

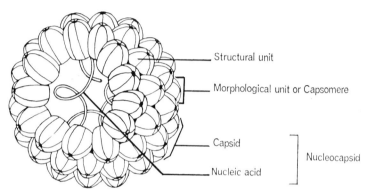

Fig. 1.1 Diagram of icosahedral virus particle with cubic symmetry. (Reproduced, with permission, from *Virus Morphology* by C.R Madeley.)

Helical — in which the particle is elongated and wound in the form of a helix or spiral; the capsomeres are arranged round the spiral of nucleic acid. Most helical viruses possess an outer envelope (Fig. 1.2).

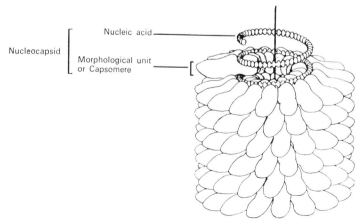

Fig. 1.2 Diagram of nucleocapsid of virus particle with helical symmetry. (Reproduced, with permission, from *Advances in Virus Research*, 1960, p. 274)

Complex — in which the particle does not confirm to either cubic or helical symmetry.

CULTIVATION OF VIRUSES

Since viruses will only replicate within living cells special methods have to be employed for culture *in vitro*; three main systems are used for cultivation of viruses in the laboratory (see Chapter 3).

1. *Tissue culture.* Cells obtained from man or animals are grown in artificial culture in glass vessels in the laboratory; these cells are living and metabolising and so can support viral replication. Most viruses can be propagated in cultures of suitable cells.
2. *Chick embryo.* Some viruses grow in the cells of the chick embryo; fertile eggs are kept in an incubator in the laboratory for this purpose. This technique has been largely superseded by tissue culture.
3. *Laboratory animals.* Before other techniques were available, viruses were isolated and studied mainly by inoculation of laboratory animals such as mice, rabbits, ferrets and monkeys; animals are still required for the isolation of a few viruses.

EFFECTS OF VIRUSES ON CELLS

Viruses may affect cells in three ways:

Cell death. The infection is lethal and kills the cell causing a cytopathic effect (CPE).

Cell transformation. The cell is not killed but is changed from a normal cell to one with the properties of a malignant or cancerous cell.

Latent infection. The virus remains within the cell in a potentially active state but produces no obvious effect on the cell's functions.

HAEMAGGLUTINATION

Although viruses cannot grow in erythrocytes, many viruses cause erythrocytes to haemagglutinate or adhere together in clumps.

CLASSIFICATION

There is as yet no entirely satisfactory classification of viruses: viruses are assigned to groups mainly on the basis of the morphology of the virus particle.

The main groups of medically-important viruses and the morphology of their particles are shown in Table 1.1.

Table 1.1 Virus classification and diseases

Family	Viruses	Diseases
DNA viruses		
Poxviruses	Variola, molluscum contagiosum	Smallpox, molluscum contagiosum
Herpesviruses	Herpes simplex, varicella-zoster, cytomegalovirus, EB virus	Herpes, chickenpox, shingles, infectious mononucleosis
Adenoviruses	Adenoviruses	Sore throats, conjunctivitis
Papovaviruses	Papilloma, polyoma, SV_{40}	Warts, progressive multifocal leucoencephalopathy
RNA viruses		
Orthomyxoviruses	Influenza	Influenza
Paramyxoviruses	Parainfluenza, respiratory syncytial, measles, mumps,	Respiratory, measles, mumps
Rhabdoviruses	Rabies	Rabies
Picornaviruses	Enteroviruses, rhinoviruses	Meningitis, poliomyelitis, colds
Togaviruses	Alphaviruses, flaviviruses	Encephalitis, febrile disease
Reoviruses	Rotavirus	Infantile diarrhoea
Arenaviruses	Lymphocytic choriomeningitis, Lassa virus	Meningitis, febrile disease

THE EFFECT OF PHYSICAL AND CHEMICAL AGENTS ON VIRUSES

Heat. Most are inactivated at 56°C for 30 minutes or at 100°C for a few seconds.

Cold. Stable at low temperatures, most can be stored at −40°C or, preferably, at −70°C; some viruses are partially inactivated by the process of freezing and thawing.

DNA Viruses

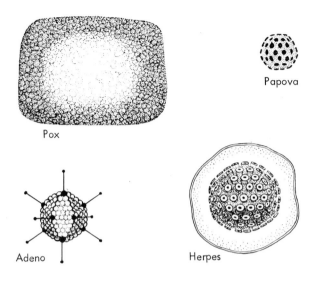

RNA Viruses

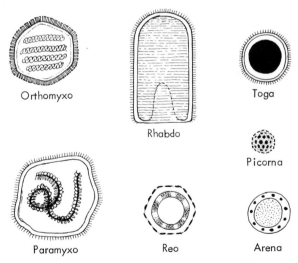

Fig. 1.3 Diagram showing the structure of the particles of different families of virus.

Drying. Variable. Some survive well, others are rapidly inactivated.

Ultra-violet irradiation. Inactivates viruses.

Chloroform and ether. Viruses with lipid-containing envelopes are inactivated, those without envelopes are resistant.

Oxidising and reducing agents. Viruses are inactivated by formaldehyde, chlorine, iodine and hydrogen peroxide.

Phenols. Most viruses are relatively resistant.

VIRUS DISEASES

Viruses are important and common causes of human disease, especially in children. Most viral infections are mild and the patient makes a complete recovery; many infections are silent and the virus multiplies in the body without causing symptoms of disease. However, viral infections which are usually mild may occasionally cause severe disease in an unusually susceptible patient; a few viral diseases are severe and always have a high mortality rate.

Entry

Viruses most often enter the body via the respiratory tract by inhalation but some viruses gain entry by ingestion, by inoculation through skin abrasions or via the bite of an arthropod vector.
Virus diseases can be of two types:
1. *Systemic.* The virus spreads widely and invades many tissues and organs as a result of viraemia or virus in the blood stream; there is a relatively long incubation period, e.g. childhood fevers such as measles and varicella.
2. *Localized.* The virus invades only tissues adjacent to the site of entry; the incubation period is usually short. Most respiratory virus infections are of this type.

Invasiveness

Virus disease is produced by direct spread of the virus to tissues and organs and not to toxin production as in bacteria. The process of virus replication in the cells of the tissues usually — but not always — kills the infected cells; this may result in lesions and disease in the tissue concerned.

HOST RESPONSE TO VIRUS INFECTION

The body defences are of two types:
(1) Non-specific
(2) Specific.

Non-specific defence mechanisms

1. *Inteferon*: probably the principal mechanism by which the body overcomes acute virus infection: interferon is a complex of protein regulatory molecules which are released from virus-infected cells; when taken up by uninfected cells these are rendered resistant to virus infection: interferon is demonstrable in blood and tissues during the acute phase of virus infections: it is host cell specific but acts against all viruses. It is of low toxicity and can be prepared (but only in small quantities) *in vitro*: it is therefore a promising anti-viral agent (see Chap. 14).
2. *Phagocytosis*: a most important defence mechanism in bacterial infection and probably in virus infections also: invading viruses — like bacteria — are ingested by two types of scavenger cell:
    (i) Neutrophil polymorphonuclear leucocytes.
    (ii) Macrophages (or mononuclear cells of the reticulo-endothelial system):
       a. free macrophages in lung alveoli, peritoneum.
       b. fixed macrophages in lymph nodes, spleen, liver (Kupffer cells), connective tissue (histiocytes) and CNS (microglia).
    Phagocytosis is enhanced by antibody (which is, of course, a specific effect) and complement: this effect is known as *opsonization*.
3. *Respiratory tract*: the constant upward movement due to the action of ciliated epithelium and the 'washing' effect of mucus.
4. *Stomach acid*: inactivates acid-labile viruses.
5. *Skin*: forms an impermeable barrier unless breached by injury, infection etc.

Specific defence mechanisms

Specific mechanisms are due to the immune system:
they are specific in that they react specifically (i.e. only) with the virus which elicited their production: the immune system has two main components:

(1) Humoral immunity (due to antibody)
(2) Cell-mediated immunity.

1. *Humoral immunity*
   Antibodies are immunoglobulins, i.e. proteins which react specifically with antigens (also usually proteins) in virus particles:
   produced by plasma cells formed when B-lymphocytes become activated after encountering antigen in spleen or lymphocytes: T-lymphocytes act as helper cells in the initial in-
   teraction between antigen and B-lymphocytes.
   Antiviral action: virus antibodies *neutralize* virus infectivity i.e.
   they render viruses non-infectious: this is an extremely effective mechanism and is responsible for the long-term immunity
   which usually follows virus infection.
   Immunoglobulins have a Y-shaped structure: the stem is the Fc
   fragment: the two arms are the Fab fragments and contain the
   antibody-combining sites: there are three main immunoglobulins which are responsible for the immune response in virus
   infection:
   (i) *IgM*: the earliest antibody produced: formed about a
       week after infection, it persists for about 4–6 weeks: a
       pentamer of five IgG molecules.
   (ii) *IgG*: formed later than IgM but persists for months and
       often years: responsible for the immunity to reinfection.
   (iii) *IgA*: a dimeric molecule: found in body secretions as
       well as blood, e.g. saliva, respiratory secretions, tears and
       intestinal contents: acquires a carbohydrate 'transport
       piece' in extracellular fluids but this is absent in serum
       IgA: the main antibody responsible for immunity to re-
       spiratory viruses and for the gut immunity seen after en-
       terovirus infection.
2. *Cell-mediated immunity*
   This, the delayed hypersensitivity response, acts to limit or
   localise the lesions of virus infections.
   T-(or thymus-dependent) lymphocytes: are the main cells involved: when sensitised or primed, T-lymphocytes react specifically with antigen and transform into blast cells with release of lymphokines.
   Lymphokines attract by chemotaxis, lymphocytes, macrophages
   and polymorphonuclear leucocytes to the site of infection.

Other factors which influence virus infection

Age
Virus infections are generally acquired in childhood and are followed by long-lasting, sometimes lifelong, immunity: a few infections of the recurrent type are more common in the elderly.

Immune deficiency

In which the host's defence mechanisms are impaired: generally results in increased susceptibility to infection: may be due to:

a. Therapy: immunosuppressive, cytoxic drugs or radiotherapy.

b. Disease: malignancy (especially leukaemia or lymphoma): some other chronic debilitating diseases: rarely, congenital immune deficiency especially that affecting cell-mediated immunity (e.g. Di George's syndrome, Swiss type hypogammaglobulinaemia).

c. Transplantation: involves deliberate immunosuppression, and impairs the host response to virus infection.

Pregnancy

Certain viruses are able to cross the placental barrier to invade the fetus: this may cause congenital abnormalities or — usually severe — infection of the fetus.

2

The biology of virus replication

Viruses show a high degree of parasitism and are metabolically inert until they infect a susceptible cell. In a susceptible cell they replicate themselves by redirecting the biochemical machinery of the cell to produce components for new virus particles; this is done by means of virus messenger RNA (mRNA).

VIRUS GROWTH CYCLE

The virus growth cycle within a cell can be divided into seven stages:

1. **Adsorption**: the first step in the invasion of a cell by virus. Some, possibly all, viruses adsorb to specific receptors on the cell plasma membrane — best at 37°C but also, although more slowly, at 4°C. Enhanced by divalent cations — Mg^{++} or Ca^{++}.

2. **Entry**: the entire virus (or sometimes only the genome) enters the cell; with many viruses the cell membrane invaginates round the adsorbed virus particle which becomes enclosed within a pinocytotic vacuole. Sometimes the virus envelope fuses with the cell membrane thus releasing the naked nucleocapsid into the cytoplasm. Uptake into the cell is temperature-dependent and takes place at 37°C but not at 4°C.

3. **Uncoating**: the protein coat of the virus is removed; this is mainly carried out by host cell enzymes contained in lysosomes. Virus nucleic acid is then released or at least made accessible for the production of virus mRNA.

4. **Transcription**: Production of virus mRNA is the key to the successful infection of the cell and is the mechanism by which a virus takes over the cellular biosynthetic machinery. Virus mRNA is made using the virus genome or nucleic acid as template (but the genome of some RNA viruses itself acts as mRNA); thus information coding for virus proteins is passed from the virus genome via virus mRNA to the cell ribosomes where the proteins are synthesised.

Structure of virus mRNA: like eukaryotic mRNA, virus mRNA molecules may contain leader sequences and are usually capped at the 5' end and polyadenylated at the 3' terminus.

Control: with many viruses, transcription of virus mRNA is complex and clearly subject to sophisticated control mechanisms. For example, the patterns of transcription are quite different in the early and late stages of the growth cycle of DNA viruses. The specificity of transcribing enzymes may play some part in this but many viruses show 'splicing' of their mRNA, i.e. the cleavage and removal from primary transcripts of sequences intervening between the expressed gene sequences.

Overlapping genes: are seen with some of the smaller DNA viruses (e.g. papovaviruses); different virus proteins are encoded by overlapping sequences in the DNA; this allows maximal use of limited coding capacity and again, points to the complexity of virus transcription.

5. **Translation**: Virus mRNA attaches to the ribosomes and directs the synthesis of *virus-specified proteins*. These are of two main types:

(i) *Structural proteins* which make up the virus particle or virion: these may be:

   a. *Capsid* proteins — closely associated with or investing the virus genome.

   b. *Envelope* proteins — glycosylated proteins which become inserted into cell membranes during replication: nucleocapsids become enveloped by budding through the modified cell plasma membrane; sometimes the envelope is acquired from the cell nuclear membrane or cytoplasmic membranes.

(ii) *Non-structural proteins* which are not incorporated into new particles. Many of these are enzymes required for the processes of virus replication (especially the synthesis of virus nucleic acid).

The number of proteins for which a virus can code is limited by the coding capacity and therefore the size of the virus genome.

6. **Assembly**: Newly synthesized nucleic acid molecules and structural proteins come together to form the particles of the new virus progeny. Depending on the virus, assembly can take place in the nucleus, the cytoplasm, or at the cell plasma membrane.

7. **Release**: The new particles are released from the cell by a gradual process of extrusion (budding) through the cell membrane or by rupture of the cell.

VIRUS GENOMES

Large viruses usually have high molecular weight nucleic acid which has the capacity to code for a large number of proteins; large viruses therefore code for many of the enzymes involved in their replication.

Small viruses have a low molecular weight nucleid acid of limited coding potential: they can therefore code for only a few proteins in addition to their structural proteins. Most use at least some of the host cell's enzymes for their replication.

Cistrons: from the point of view of genetic functions, the virus genome can be sub-divided into cistrons each of which contains the information to code for one functional polypeptide or protein.

Table 2.1 gives examples of the main virus groups with details about some properties of their genome.

BIOCHEMISTRY OF VIRUS REPLICATION

The biochemical processes involved in virus replication are directed to the synthesis of virus proteins and nucleic acid genomes. Clearly DNA and RNA viruses must differ in the mechanisms involved. Below are brief descriptions of the replication of selected examples of the principal types of pathogenic virus:

DNA viruses

Examples: Vaccinia, herpes simplex, adenovirus, papovaviruses.

Almost all pathogenic DNA viruses contain double-stranded DNA so that although single-stranded DNA viruses exist, they will not be described here. The principal stages in the replication of a double-stranded DNA virus are shown diagrammatically in Figure 2.1.

Initial stage: After entry to the cell, the virus DNA becomes uncoated. Vaccinia virus, however, is unusual and uncoats in two stages — the first by host cell enzymes which allows some limited early transcription to take place: this results in production of a virus-coded protein which then completes the uncoating process. After release from its capsid, the virus genome acts as a template for synthesis of virus mRNA.

Table 2.1 Some properties of viruses and their genomes

Virus	Nucleic acid Type[a]	Nucleic acid Molecular weight ($\times 10^6$ daltons)	Infectivity	Transcriptase contained in virus particles	Number of virion structural proteins
Vaccinia	DS DNA	120	0	+	48
Herpes simplex	DS DNA	100	+	0	30
Adenovirus	DS DNA	23	+	0	14
Polyoma	DS DNA	3	+	0	3
Poliovirus	SS RNA	2.6	+	0	5
Sindbis (a togavirus)	SS RNA	3.5	+	0	3
Influenza A	SS RNA[c]	5.7	0	+	7
Parainfluenza	SS RNA	5	0	+	6
Rous sarcoma	SS RNA	10	0	+[b]	7
Reovirus	DS RNA[c]	15	0	+	7

Modified and reproduced, with permission, from a table originally drawn up by Dr C.R. Pringle
a DS = double-stranded; SS = single-stranded
b reverse transcriptase
c fragmented

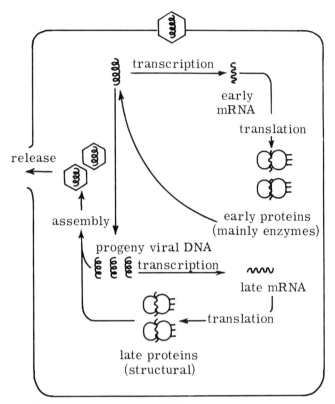

Fig. 2.1 Diagram of replicative cycle of DNA virus.

Transcription: takes place in two stages:
1. *Early*: before virus DNA synthesis: early virus mRNA codes mainly for the enzymes required for virus DNA synthesis; host cell DNA, RNA and protein synthesis are halted at this stage.
2. *Late*: after the onset of DNA synthesis; late virus mRNA codes mainly for virus structural proteins.

Virus DNA synthesis: many enzymes are involved in this but the most important is DNA-dependent DNA polymerase. This enzyme may be coded by:
1. the host cell (adenovirus, papovavirus)
2. the virus (vaccinia, herpes simplex viruses): produced from early mRNA.

Note: vaccinia and herpes simplex viruses code for some of the other enzymes involved in DNA synthesis (e.g. deoxypyrimidine kinase).

Template: the DNA genome of the parental virus is the template for the synthesis of progeny DNA molecules.

Timing: virus DNA synthesis takes place at the end of the early phase of the virus growth cycle.

New virus DNA: the progeny DNA molecules act as templates for the transcription of late virus mRNA as well as genomes for new virus particles.

Virus protein synthesis: the majority — but not all — structural proteins are synthesized from late mRNA: some are coded by early mRNA. Protein synthesis especially with the larger DNA viruses like vaccinia and herpes simplex, is subject to complex controls. For example, the timing and quantity of the synthesis of individual proteins varies throughout the growth cell: some viruses show cascade regulation in which synthesis of early proteins is necessary for the 'switch-on' of later proteins.

Site: virus proteins are synthesized on cell ribosomes in the cytoplasm and transported from there to the site of assembly: translation involves host cell transfer RNA species.

Assembly: the assembly (or morphogenesis) of virus progeny particles from newly synthesized virus proteins and DNA molecules may take place in:
1. *Nucleus*: (herpes simplex, adenovirus, papovaviruses) Proteins synthesized in the cytoplasm are transported to the nucleus where, with virus DNA molecules, they are assembled into the nucleocapsids of new virus particles: the particles of herpes simplex virus acquire an envelope by budding through the nuclear membrane (which is modified by the incorporation within it of virus glycoproteins).
2. *Cytoplasm*: (vaccinia virus) vaccinia virus replicates entirely in the cytoplasm in 'factories' which are clusters of ribosomes where both virus protein and DNA synthesis take place.

RNA Viruses
Because their genetic material is RNA instead of DNA, RNA viruses are of great biological interest. Clearly, their replication must involve radically different mechanisms from those involved in DNA virus replication. For example, the necessity to use RNA as template instead of the usual DNA implies that enzymes will be re-

quired which are unlikely to be found in uninfected cells. Such enzymes would therefore have to be virus-coded.

mRNA: like DNA viruses, the crucial factor in the successful infection of a cell is the production of virus mRNA.

RNA viruses are divided into two groups depending on the nature of their RNA genome:

1. *Positive-strand* viruses in which the input RNA genome acts as mRNA; these RNA genomes are infectious and when applied to cells the purified RNA can initiate a complete infectious cycle of virus replication.
2. *Negative-strand* viruses in which the input virus RNA genome is transcribed into mRNA. RNA viruses of this sort contain a transcriptase or RNA-dependent RNA polymerase within their particle; since the transcriptase is essential for infectivity, the purified RNA genome is not infectious.

Positive-strand RNA viruses

Example: poliovirus

The principal steps in the multiplication of positive-strand RNA viruses are illustrated diagrammatically in Figure 2.2

Transcription: After uncoating, the RNA genome of the infecting particle functions as virus mRNA and attaches to host cell ribosomes for translation into virus-specified proteins; poliovirus RNA is polycistronic, i.e. it codes for a single very large polypeptide.

Virus RNA synthesis: Progeny RNA molecules are replicated by a virus-coded enzyme — RNA-dependent RNA polymerase: this enzyme is produced by cleavage from the large polypeptide which is the primary product of transcription. Virus RNA synthesis takes place in the following stages:

1. A second negative RNA strand which is complementary to the input positive RNA genome is produced with formation of a double-stranded RNA structure known as the replicative form.
2. New positive RNA strands are synthesized using as template the complementary negative RNA strand of the double-stranded replicative form.

The new progeny (positive-strand) RNA molecules have three functions:

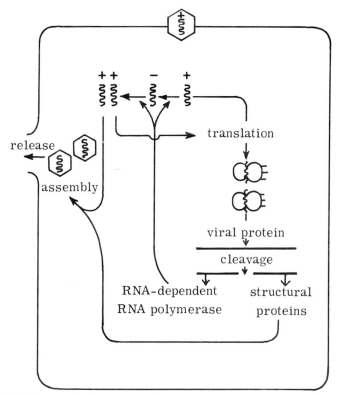

Fig. 2.2 Diagram of replicative cycle of plus-strand RNA virus.

1. *Templates* for the manufacture of more replicative forms for further synthesis of RNA genomes.
2. *Genomes* for new virus particles: RNA molecules which become genomes in new virus particles have a small protein linked to their 5′ termini.
3. *Virus mRNA*: the newly synthesized RNA which acts as mRNA does not become encapsidated as the genomes of new particles.

Translation

With positive strand RNA viruses, virus mRNA is translated into a single very large polypeptide: the individual virus proteins — both structural and non-structural — are then produced from this large protein by cleavage due to the action of virus-coded proteolytic enzymes. The cleavage is a complex process and takes place in several stages. The proteins finally produced include RNA-dependent RNA polymerase and four capsid proteins.

Assembly: poliovirus replicates and new progeny virus particles are assembled on clusters of ribosomes in the cytoplasm: the new progeny particles are released by sudden rupture of the cell.

Negative-strand RNA viruses

Examples: influenza, parainfluenza viruses.

The principal stages in the replication of this type of virus are shown diagrammatically in Figure 2.3.

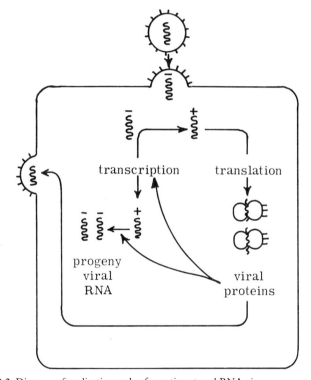

Fig. 2.3 Diagram of replicative cycle of negative-strand RNA virus.

Initial stages: These viruses are enveloped and enter cells by fusion of their envelope with the cell plasma membrane — the nucleocapsid thereby becoming released into the cytoplasm.

Transcription and virus RNA synthesis: particles of negative-strand RNA viruses contain a RNA-dependent RNA polymerase: this enzyme transcribes in two stages:
1. Parental negative RNA strands are transcribed into positive

RNA strands which in turn act as templates for the synthesis of negative strand RNA genomes for incorporation into new virus particles.
2. Positive RNA strands are synthesised to act, not as templates for new genomes, but as mRNA molecules. After transcription, individual mRNA molecules corresponding to each virus protein are cleaved from the large primary RNA transcript.

Note: the influenza virus genome consists of 8 RNA fragments each of which codes for a different virus protein. Influenza virus is unusual amongst these viruses in that its multiplication requires transcription of host cell DNA — possibly because cellular mRNAs act as primers for virus RNA synthesis.

Virus protein synthesis: virus proteins are produced on ribosomes in the cell cytoplasm. The proteins include nucleocapsid proteins, the transcriptase (RNA-dependent RNA polymerase), a matrix protein, and two glycosylated envelope proteins — the haemagglutinin and neuraminidase. The two glycoproteins form the characteristic spikes seen in the envelope of virus particles on electron microscopy. The haemagglutinin protein requires to be cleaved (a process carried out by host cell enzymes) for infectivity: in cells lacking the appropriate enzyme, the virus particles are non-infectious.

Assembly: most negative strand RNA viruses are assembled at the cell plasma membrane: virus glycoproteins become inserted into the membrane and nucleocapsids formed just below the cell margin become enveloped — and released — by budding through the altered cell membrane. Influenza virus is an exception; its nucleocapsids are formed in the cell nucleus.

Replication of RNA tumour viruses

Example: Rous sarcoma virus.

RNA tumour viruses (now classified as retroviruses) not only replicate in cells but can transform cells into malignant or cancer cells. They have an unusual mode of replication which reflects their oncogenic or tumour-producing properties. Their replication is shown diagrammatically in Figure 2.4.

Structure: RNA tumour viruses have enveloped particles with a nucleoprotein core which contains single-stranded RNA. The particles contain a unique enzyme — reverse transcriptase (RNA-

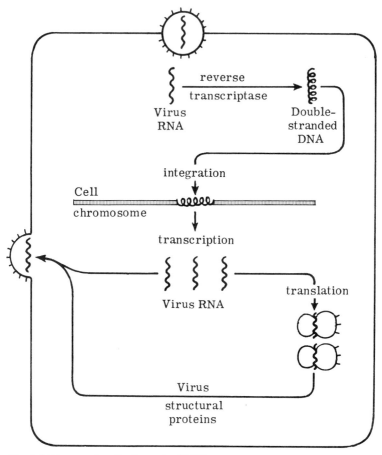

Fig. 2.4 Diagram of replicative cycle of RNA tumour virus.

dependent DNA polymerase). Their genome consists of two identical RNA molecules hydrogen-bonded near their 5′ termini each of
which has an associated molecule of tryptophan transfer RNA.
They contain four genes which code for the following proteins:

gag   (core proteins)
pol   (polymerase — the reverse transcriptase)
env   (envelope glycoproteins)
onc   (the transforming protein — a protein kinase)

Transcription: there are two phases:
1. *First*: on infection of a cell, the particle-associated reverse transcriptase directs the synthesis of a virus-specific single-stranded

DNA molecule off the parental RNA genome. The same enzyme then converts the single-stranded molecule into linear double-stranded DNA.

Integration: the double-stranded DNA molecule (which contains all the virus information transcribed from the parental RNA) then integrates into the cell chromosome. It is then known as a *provirus*.

2. *Second*: The second phase of transcription is carried out by host cell enzymes and transcribes the integrated provirus DNA copy in the chromosome. Different kinds of transcript are produced:

 (i) Full-length transcripts of RNA for encapsidation as genomes in new virus particles.

 (ii) Shorter transcripts of mRNA from the *gag* gene with occasional read-through of the *pol* gene: this results in the synthesis of more *gag* gene product then polymerase (much less transcriptase than core proteins is required for incorporation into new particles).

 (iii) Full-length transcripts of mRNA in which the sequences for the *gag* and *pol* are spliced out to yield mRNA for the *env* gene.

 (iv) *onc* gene mRNA produced from a transcript in which *gag*, *pol* and *env* gene sequences are spliced out.

Virus protein synthesis: the *gag* gene product is a large protein which is cleaved (probably by a virus-coded protein) to form four core proteins. The *env* gene product is a glycoprotein and this is cleaved into two glycoproteins which form the spikes seen in the virus envelope on electron microscopy.

Transformation: The *onc* — or transforming gene — codes for a protein kinase: it is probably originally a cellular gene that has become integrated into the virus genome: the protein enzyme it encodes phosphorylates tyrosine residues.

Assembly: takes place at the cell surface: nucleocapsids assemble beneath the cell membrane and acquire their envelope by budding through the membrane modified by the insertion into it of the two virus glycoproteins.

3

Laboratory diagnosis of virus infection

Virus diseases are diagnosed by:
1. **Isolation** of virus.
2. **Direct demonstration** of virus or antigen in material from the patient.
3. **Serology**, i.e. demonstration of virus antibody.

ISOLATION

Virus isolation requires the use of living cells since viruses cannot grow on inanimate media. There are three main systems:
1. Tissue culture
2. Chick embryo
3. Laboratory animals.

Note: Almost all virus isolation is nowadays done in tissue culture.

1. TISSUE CULTURE

Tissue culture is really cell culture and consists of the preparation of a single layer (monolayer) of actively metabolising cells adherent to a glass or plastic surface in a test tube, petri plate or on one side of a flat bottle.
The main types of tissue culture are:
1. *Primary cultures*: laborious to prepare and shortlived but generally susceptible to a wide range of viruses. Prepared by trypsinising fresh tissue to disperse the cells which are then seeded into suitable culture vessels. There is little cell division and although one subculture can be done, the cells die in about two to three weeks, e.g. rhesus monkey kidney (now difficult to obtain in quantity) and human amnion.
2. *Semi-continuous cell strains*: are established from human embryo lung. easy to maintain and can be subcultured for about 30 to 40

passages before the cells die off. Susceptible to a wide range of viruses.

3. *Continuous cell lines*: (can be subcultured indefinitely and are therefore easy to maintain.) Generally susceptible to fewer viruses than the other types of cell culture. HeLa (derived from human cervical cancer) is the most widely known but is less useful for virus isolation than the newly introduced RD cell line of human rhabdomyosarcoma.

Medium: cells are grown in chemically defined media which are balanced and buffered salt solutions with added amino acids and vitamins. Serum is always required — generally 10% (by volume) of calf serum (or sometimes fetal calf serum for delicate cells). Penicillin and streptomycin are included to prevent bacterial contamination.

Atmosphere: because the main buffer in the medium is bicarbonate, cells produce carbon dioxide: if this is lost to the air, e.g. in open petri plates, the pH of the medium becomes alkaline and kills the cells. Tissue cultures are therefore often grown in closed vessels, e.g. test tubes stoppered with rubber bungs or screw-capped bottles. Petri plates or test tubes with cotton wool plugs or loose metal caps must be incubated in an atmosphere enriched with 5 to 10% carbon dioxide.

Temperature: the optimal temperature is 37°C.

Specimens

Material from lesions or sites of infection usually collected on a wooden-shafted swab. The tip of the swab is broken off into a bottle of transport medium. Virus laboratories supply these on request.

Delivery: should be prompt as many viruses die off rapidly at room temperature. If delay is unavoidable, keep the specimen at 4°C (e.g. in a domestic refrigerator).

Inoculation: the method of inoculation is shown in Figure 3.1

Virus growth is recognised by:
1. *CPE* (cytopathic effect): the virus kills the cells which round up and fall off the glass (see Figs 3.1 and 3.2). Some viruses cause

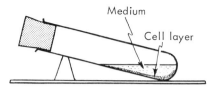

Test tube containing tissue culture:
incubated in slightly tilted position so that
cells settle and grow up one side of tube.

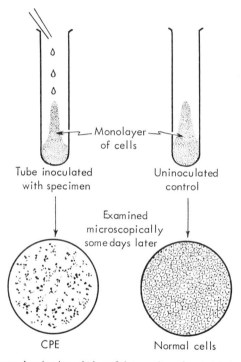

Fig. 3.1 Diagram showing inoculation of tissue culture for viral isolation.

cell fusion and their growth is recognised by the appearance of syncytia.

2. *Haemadsorption*: added erythrocytes adhere to the surface of infected cells. Seen with haemagglutinating viruses because the haemagglutinin protein appears in the cell plasma membrane and projects from it.

3. *Immunofluorescence*: infected cells are detected by fluorescence when virus antibody which has been tagged with fluorescent dye is added to the cell culture.

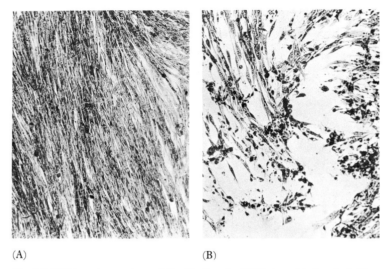

(A)   (B)

Fig. 3.2 CPE in a tissue culture of fibroblastic cells. (A) Uninoculated control. (B) Culture showing viral CPE.

Identification of virus isolates: is usually done by serology:

1. *Neutralization test*: the infectivity of the virus (i.e. its CPE) is neutralized by antibody. The isolate is tested against various standard antisera and the one which neutralizes its infectivity identifies it.

   Example

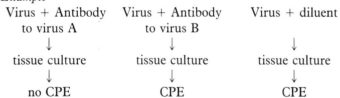

   Virus + Antibody   Virus + Antibody   Virus + diluent
      to virus A   to virus B
          ↓   ↓   ↓
   tissue culture   tissue culture   tissue culture
          ↓   ↓   ↓
       no CPE   CPE   CPE

   The virus is therefore identified as virus A.

2. *Haemagglutination-inhibition*: haemadsorbing viruses are identified by harvesting the virus and testing it for inhibition by standard antiviral sera of its ability to haemagglutinate (see p. 29).

3. *Immunofluorescence*: a specific immunological test which, if used to detect virus in tissue cultures, has the great advantage that it simultaneously identifies the virus serologically.

4. *Electron microscopy*: occasionally useful for the rapid detection of characteristic virus particles in the tissue culture.

2. CHICK EMBRYO

Rarely used nowadays. Figure 3.3 shows the main routes of inoculation.

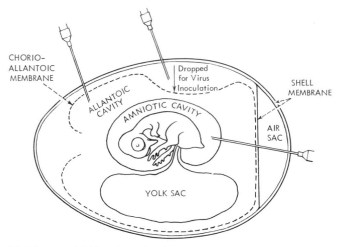

Fig. 3.3 Diagram of chick embryo showing routes of inoculation for viral isolation.

Virus growth is recognised by the appearance of (i) pocks (or virus lesions) on the chorio-allantoic membrane or (ii) haemagglutinin in the amniotic or allantoic fluids (see Fig. 3.4)

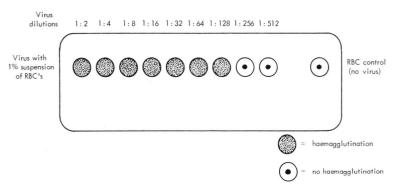

Fig. 3.4 Diagram of haemagglutination test for virus. Titre of virus haemagglutinin is 128.

Identification of virus is serological e.g. by testing for pock reduction or haemagglutination-inhibition with standard antiviral sera.

3. LABORATORY ANIMALS

Some viruses can only be isolated by inoculation of laboratory animals, usually mice. After inoculation the animals are observed for signs of disease or death. The viruses are identified by testing for neutralization of their pathogenicity for animals by standard antiviral sera.

DIRECT DEMONSTRATION OF VIRUS

Now becoming a widely used — and fast — method of virus diagnosis. Virus or virus antigen is detected in lesions, fluids, tissues or excretions from the patient and a result can be obtained within an hour or two of receipt of the specimen. The main techniques are:

1. *Serological*: the most popular is immunofluorescence; enzyme immunoassay and radioimmune assay are now also being used for this.
2. *Electron microscopy*: virus particles are detected and can be provisionally identified (but not serologically typed) on the basis of their morphology.

Inclusion bodies — are virus-induced masses seen in the nucleus or cytoplasm of infected cells. With a few exceptions they are too non-specific to be useful in diagnosis.

SEROLOGY

Detection of antibody is by far the most widely used method of virological diagnosis. However, virus antibodies are common in healthy populations and recent infection can only be diagnosed by the following criteria:

1. *Rising titre*: i.e. increase in the level of virus antibody at least four-fold over the course of the illness and into convalescence. A four-fold rise in antibody titre is incontrovertible evidence of recent virus infection.
   (*Note*: titre is the highest dilution of an antiserum at which activity can be demonstrated: it is expressed as the reciprocal of the dilution, i.e. 64 rather than 1/64).
2. *Detection of IgM*: IgM — the earliest antibody to appear — is only present if there has been recent infection with the virus. Tests for virus-specific IgM are now becoming widely used in virus laboratories.

3. *High stationary titre*: if the level of virus antibody is *considerably* higher than that found in the general population, recent infection with the virus can be assumed. Because of the great variation in antibody levels in normal people this is a less reliable method of diagnosis.

SEROLOGICAL TESTS

Increasingly tests are being developed to detect antibody in a single serum sample taken in the acute stage of the disease. Traditionally virus diagnosis depended on the demonstration of a rise in titre in two blood samples — one taken in the acute illness and one ten to fourteen days later. There are many techniques for the detection of virus antibody. Below are brief descriptions of those most often used:

1. **Complement fixation test:** the most widely used test but generally not very sensitive. Tests are carried out in two stages:
   (i) Dilutions of the serum under test are mixed with virus and complement overnight at 4°.
   (ii) An indicator system (sheep erythrocytes sensitized with anti-sheep erythrocyte antibody) is added the following morning at 37° to detect the presence of complement.
   If complement has been fixed in Stage (i) (i.e. the patient's serum contained antibody) there is no haemolysis of the sheep erythrocytes. Haemolysis indicates that there was no

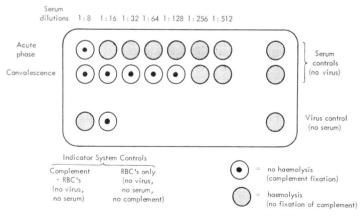

Fig. 3.5 Diagram of complement-fixation test for viral antibody. Virus antigen is mixed overnight at 4°C with dilutions of the patient's serum and complement before addition of sensitised sheep erythrocytes. Titre of complement-fixing antibody has risen from 8 in the acute phase to 128 in convalescene — a greater than 4-fold rise in titre indicating recent infection.

antibody in the patient's serum. A simplified complement fixation test is illustrated diagrammatically in Figure 3.5.

2. **Immunofluorescence**: Fluorescent antibody tests are widely used in virology — most often by the sandwich or indirect test. In this, dilutions of patient's serum are added to spots of virus-infected cells on microscope slides. After washing, virus antibody is detected by the subsequent application of fluorescein-labelled anti-human IgG. Fluorescence is seen by examination in a microscope under ultra-violet light; it indicates the presence of virus antibody and — according to the highest dilution at which this is observed — the titre of antibody.

    Note: by using anti-human IgM as the fluorescein-labelled antibody, virus specific IgM can be detected (see p. 30).

3. **Haemagglutination-inhibition**: antibody to haemagglutinating viruses can be measured by testing for the ability of patient's serum to inhibit virus haemagglutination (see Fig. 3.6). Although the test itself is relatively simple to perform, the frequency of non-specific inhibitors of haemagglutination in normal serum means that preliminary absorption to remove these has often to be carried out.

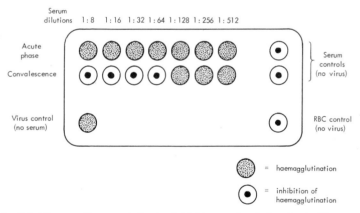

Fig. 3.6 Diagram of haemagglutination-inhibition test for viral antibody. The haemagglutinating virus is mixed with dilutions of the patient's serum for one hour before addition of erythrocytes. Titre of haemagglutination-inhibiting antibody has risen from less than 8 in the acute phase to 64 in convalescence — a greater than 4-fold rise in titre indicating recent infection.

Radial immune haemolysis: is a related but qualitative method of detecting antibody to haemagglutinating viruses. Suitable erythrocytes are coated with virus and incorporated together with complement into an agar gel in a plastic plate. Patients' sera are then added to wells cut in the agar. After incubation, the presence of antibody is detected by the appearance of zones of haemolysis round the wells. The titre of antibody cannot be measured by this test: it is only useful for detecting the presence or absence of antibody in a sample and cannot be used to diagnose active infection. Its main use is to screen normal people for immunity to a virus and therefore to indicate those who may require vaccination.

4. **Neutralization test**: dilutions of patient's serum are tested for their ability to neutralize a standard virus preparation. This is the converse of the other application of neutralization tests, i.e. when an unknown virus is identified by testing for neutralization with known (or standard) antivirus antibody (see p. 25).

5. **Enzyme-immuno-assay (EIA)**: an extremely sensitive method of detecting virus antibody. Similar in principle to immunofluorescence but the anti-human IgG antibody is tagged with an enzyme which reacts when a suitable substrate is later added to produce a visible colour change. The enzyme-substrate combinations most often used are horseradish peroxidase and hydrogen peroxide acting on orthophenyl-diamine and alkaline phosphatase acting on para-nitrophenyl phosphate: both reactions produce a yellow colour. Probably the principal virus serological test of the future.

6. **Radio-immune assay (RIA)**: generally the most sensitive technique and also similar in principle to immunofluorescence. The anti-human IgG antibody is in this instance tagged with a radioactive isotope — most often I^{125}. The disadvantages of the test are the problems of organising a laboratory for radioactive work, expense and the fact that the radioactive conjugates have a limited shelf life.

7. **Detection of IgM** can be done in two ways:
   (i) *Serologically*: patient's serum is reacted with virus antigen (usually virus-infected cells fixed on a slide). IgM antibody is then detected by application of anti-human IgM antibody labelled either with fluorescein, radio-isotope (e.g. I^{125}) or enzyme (i.e. EIA). Attachment of the labelled antibody to the virus complex indicates the presence of virus-specific IgM.
   (ii) *Physically*: IgM can be separated from IgG in patient's serum by centrifugation in a sucrose density gradient; the IgM fraction is then tested for antiviral antibody by standard techniques.

4

Influenza

Influenza is one of the great epidemic diseases. From time to time, influenza becomes pandemic and sweeps throughout the world. The most severe pandemic recorded was in the winter of 1918 to 1919, when more than 20 million people perished. World-wide pandemics of influenza are due to the emergence of antigenically new strains of influenza virus to which there is no pre-existing immunity.

Clinical features

Route of infections
Inhalation of respiratory secretions from an infected person.

Incubation period
From 1 to 4 days.

Signs and symptoms
Fever, malaise, headache, generalized aches, sometimes with nasal discharge and sneezing; a non-productive hacking cough is common and there may be sore throat and hoarseness.

Duration
Symptoms usually last for about 4 days but tiredness and weakness often persist for longer.

Primary site of virus multiplication
Superficial epithelium of the upper and lower respiratory tract; influenza causes damage to the cilia and desquamation of the epithelium.

Complications
In a small proportion of cases, the acute infection progresses to pneumonia: two kinds of pneumonia may follow influenza:

1. *Primary influenzal pneumonia*, in which the condition of a patient with typical influenza suddenly deteriorates with the onset of severe respiratory distress and symptoms of hypoxia, dyspnoea and cyanosis; circulatory collapse follows and in most cases the patient dies. *Post mortem*, there is congestion of the lungs with desquamation of ciliated epithelium and hyperaemia of tracheal and bronchial mucosa; no significant bacteria are present.

2. *Secondary bacterial pneumonia*, usually develops later in the course of influenza and is due to secondary invasion of the lungs by bacteria such as *Staphylococcus aureus*, *Haemophilus influenzae* or pneumococci. The signs and symptoms are those of severe bacterial pneumonia; although there is a high mortality rate, the disease is less lethal than primary influenzal pneumonia. *Post mortem* there is heavy invasion of the lungs by bacteria.

Reye's syndrome
This is a rare complication mainly seen after influenza B in children; there is cerebral oedema and fatty degeneration of the viscera — especially the liver — which results in raised transaminase levels in the blood; there is a high mortality rate.

Types of virus
There are three influenza viruses, A, B and C, which can be differentiated by complement fixation test:
   A — the principal cause of epidemic influenza;
   B — usually associated with a milder disease but can also cause winter epidemics;
   C — of doubtful pathogenicity for man.
   Influenza A viruses are also found in animals — notably birds, pigs, and horses.

Epidemiology

Seasonal distribution
The highest incidence of infection is during the winter (but the epidemic of 'Asian' influenza started in Britain in the summer of 1957).

Spread
This is more rapid than in any other infectious disease: in addition to other important properties, influenza virus possesses an inherent capacity for rapid spread.

Epidemics

Pandemics of influenza A break out every few years and the epidemic strain spreads world-wide. The most severe epidemic with a high mortality rate was in 1918–19 and was due to a virus related to swine influenza A virus; unlike most influenza outbreaks, there was a relatively high mortality amongst young adults: usually influenza is most severe in the elderly or in patients with chronic respiratory or cardiac disease.

Virology

1. Orthomyxoviruses ('myxo' = affinity for mucin).
2. RNA viruses — the RNA consists of eight separate fragments each of which codes for a different protein, e.g. the haemagglutinin, the neuraminidase. etc.
3. Roughly spherical particles, medium size, 80 to 100 nm, with an envelope which contains radially-projecting spikes of virus haemagglutinin and neuraminidase; inside the envelope is helically coiled ribonucleoprotein (Fig. 4.1).
4. Haemagglutinate erythrocytes of various animal species.
5. Grow in amniotic cavity of the chick embryo and — after passage or subculture — in the allantoic cavity also.
6. Grow in monkey kidney tissue culture with haemadsorption.

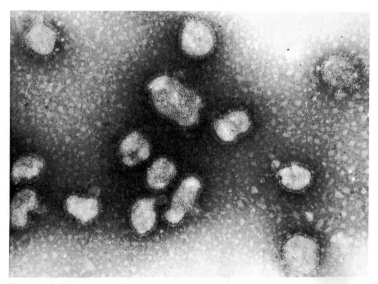

Fig. 4.1 Influenza virus. The virus nucleocapsid (or nucleic acid with protein capsid) has helical symmetry and is surrounded by an envelope containing spikes of haemagglutinin and neuraminidase × 90 000. (Photograph by Dr E.A.C. Follett.)

HAEMAGGLUTINATION BY INFLUENZA VIRUSES

Haemagglutination is due to adsorption of influenza virus particles to specific receptors on the erythrocyte surface.

Receptors are composed of muco-polysaccharide — neuraminic acid.

Virus haemagglutinin is contained on the radially-projecting spikes in the envelope round the virus particle; the haemagglutinin has a combining site which is antigenic and has an affinity for neuraminic acid.

Neuraminidase. Influenza virus particles also contain an enzyme which is similar in action to the receptor destroying enzyme (RDE) of *Vibrio cholerae*; this destroys the neuraminic acid receptors on erythrocytes. After viral haemagglutination, if the mixture of virus and erythrocytes is kept at 37°C, the neuraminidase causes the virus to elute from the erythrocytes; as a result the haemagglutination is reversed and the erythrocytes disperse again.

Haemagglutination-inhibition. Treatment of the virus with specific antibody prevents haemagglutination. Haemagglutination-inhibition is strain-specific, i.e. haemagglutination by a new virus strain, is unaffected by antibody to an influenza virus strain with a different haemagglutinin.

ANTIGENIC STRUCTURE

Influenza viruses have three main antigens:
1. '*S*' *or soluble antigen* — the protein in the ribonucleoprotein core of the virus particle: this antigen is type specific in that all influenza A viruses share a common S antigen which is different to that shared by all influenza B viruses; demonstrated by complement fixation test.
2. *Haemagglutinin*: contained in the radially-projecting spikes in the virus envelope; strain-specific; the main neutralising antigen responsible for immunity to the virus.
3. *Neuraminidase*: the enzyme also contained in the virus envelope; plays a minor role in immunity to reinfection.

Antigenic variation
Influenza viruses are unusual among viruses in that they undergo

antigenic change from time to time. Epidemics are due to the emergence of a new virus strain containing a haemagglutinin or neuraminidase that differs from those in previously circulating viruses either completely (*antigenic shift*) or partially (*antigenic drift*). Epidemics arise because the population has no herd immunity (i.e. antibody) to the new haemagglutinin.

Antigenic shift is illustrated by the serological types of haemagglutinin and neuraminidase contained in the major influenza virus A strains which have circulated in the world during the past 40 years or so:

Virus strain	Haemagglutinin	Neuraminidase
A/FM/1/47	H1	N1
A/Singapore/1/57	H2	N2
A/Hong Kong/1/68	H3	N2

Note: the last two digits in the designation of the virus strain refer to the year when it was first isolated.

Genetic recombination: because of its fragmented genome, influenza virus shows a high rate of recombination or genetic reassortment during replication. There is evidence that new human strains of influenza virus A can arise by recombination with avian and animal strains of influenza virus A; as a result, a new virus emerges which has acquired, by recombination, genetic material which codes for a new haemagglutinin or neuraminidase and which has been derived from an animal virus strain.

Antigenic shift takes place every 10 to 15 years. This involves the replacement of the main neutralizing antigen — the haemagglutinin — by a different protein acquired as a result of genetic reassortment when the appropriate RNA segment which codes for the haemagglutinin is exchanged in the virus genome for one from another source.

Several pandemics of influenza have been recorded this century:
1. 1918–19: almost certainly due to a virus of which the haemagglutinin was similar to one commonly found in swine influenza strains.
2. 1934: the first influenza virus was isolated.
3. 1947: H1N1 virus emerged.
4. 1957: H2N2 — the 'Asian flu' epidemic.
5. 1968: H3N2 — the 'Hong Kong flu' epidemic.

6. 1977: H1N1 reappeared — 'Red flu' — but caused infection only in young people under 20 years of age — older people having antibody from exposure to the virus in 1947–1957.

At present: both H3N2 and H1N1 strains have circulated together in countries throughout the world since 1977 and did so in the winter 1980–81: in 1981–82, in Britain, only H3N2 caused infection.

Antigenic drift is due to a minor change in the amino acid sequence of the haemagglutinin protein but the haemagglutinin remains basically the same protein. The changes are the result of spontaneous mutations; the mutant strains of virus then become selected in the population by their ability to infect partially immune hosts: antigenic drift increases progressively from season to season.

Influenza B

Also shows antigenic variation but the changes are less dramatic than with influenza A.
1. 1973: a new strain B/Hong Kong/5/73 appeared.
2. 1979: B/Singapore/222/79 appeared.

At present: circulating strains show considerable heterogeneity but generally resemble the 1979 virus more closely than the 1973 strain.

Diagnosis

Isolation

Specimens: mouth washings and throat swabs

Inoculate:
1. Monkey kidney tissue cultures
   Observe for haemagglutination or hacmadsorption of human group O erythrocytes.
   Virus is typed by haemagglutination-inhibition with specific antisera.
2. Amniotic cavity of chick embryo
   Observe for haemagglutination of fowl erythrocytes.
   Virus is typed by testing for inhibition of haemagglutination with standard antisera.

Serology

Complement fixation test: with the 'S' or soluble antigen

Haemagglutination-inhibition test. The reaction is strain-specific, so tests must be done with currently circulating strains of virus.

Vaccines

Because of the considerable morbidity and the risk of fatal complications, vaccines have been developed against influenza viruses.

At the time of a pandemic, the speed with which new strains of influenza virus spread makes it difficult if not impossible to prepare sufficient quantities of vaccine in time to protect any but a few key workers.

There are two types of influenza vaccine:

Inactivated virus vaccines

Administered by subcutaneous injection; saline suspension of purified virus grown in the allantoic cavity of the chick embryo or virus subunits (i.e. haemagglutinin and neuraminidase)

In general, influenza vaccines give relatively short-lived immunity — usually lasting only a few months. At best the protection conferred is of the order of 60 per cent.

Guillain-Barré syndrome: a polyneuritis with ascending paralysis usually starting in the legs has been reported as a significant complication following the mass influenza vaccine campaign in the USA during the winter of 1976–77. The disease usually clears up spontaneously although occasionally positive pressure respiration is required during the acute phase due to paralysis of the respiratory muscles.

Live attenuated virus vaccines

Administered intra-nasally but live vaccines have not become generally accepted.

5

Upper respiratory tract infections

The vast majority of viral respiratory infections primarily involve the upper respiratory tract. In fact, the classification of respiratory tract infections as 'upper' or 'lower' is only partially correct as most respiratory viruses can and do infect both upper and lower respiratory tracts. Upper respiratory syndromes often show some involvement of the lower respiratory tract and vice versa.

Respiratory infections are a major problem in medicine because of their frequency: they are also of considerable economic importance because they cause so much absence from work. So far, there is no foreseeable prospect of controlling these infections; most spread rapidly by inhalation of infected respiratory secretions.

The main viruses which affect the upper respiratory tract are shown in Table 5.1.

Table 5.1 Viruses which affect the upper respiratory tract

Virus	No. of serotypes	Disease
Parainfluenza viruses	4	croup; colds, lower respiratory infections in children
Respiratory syncytial virus	1	bronchiolitis and pneumonia in infants, colds in older children
Rhinoviruses	100+	colds
Adenoviruses	33	pharyngitis and conjunctivitis
Coronaviruses	3	colds
Coxsackieviruses	types A21, B3	colds
Echoviruses	types 11, 20	colds

PARAINFLUENZA VIRUSES

Clinical features

Most common syndrome: associated with parainfluenza viruses is febrile common cold with sore throat, hoarseness and cough.

38

Croup is an acute laryngo-tracheobronchitis characterized by hoarseness and cough; in infants, the disease may be very severe with respiratory distress, inspiratory stridor and cyanosis requiring tracheostomy.

Bronchiolitis and pneumonia in young children are also sometimes caused by parainfluenza viruses.

Age. The viruses affect both children and adults but infection is most common in children under 5 years old; the more severe parainfluenza lower respiratory tract infections are seen mainly in these pre-school children.

Serotypes. There are 4 parainfluenza viruses — types 1, 2, 3 and 4 — but type 4 is of low pathogenicity.

Serotypes and disease. Although there is considerable overlap, type 3 virus is particularly associated with bronchiolitis and bronchopneumonia and types 1 and 2 with croup.

Epidemiology. Type 3 infects younger children than types 1 and 2 and more often affects the lower respiratory tract: it causes outbreaks of infection every year; type 1 outbreaks in contrast are seen every 2 years.

Virology
1. Paramyxoviruses.
2. RNA viruses.
3. Large enveloped particles, 100 to 200 nm, with helical symmetry possessing both a haemagglutinin and a neuraminidase.
4. Haemagglutinate human group O erythrocytes.
5. Grow in monkey kidney tissue cultures with haemadsorption.

Diagnosis

Isolation

Specimens: mouth washings, throat swabs.

Inoculate: monkey kidney tissue cultures.

Observe: for haemadsorption with human group O erythrocytes (CPE is variable and slow).

Type virus: by neutralisation test of haemadsorption by standard antisera.

Serology
Complement fixation test.

RESPIRATORY SYNCYTIAL VIRUS

Respiratory syncytial virus causes common colds but its importance lies in its tendency to invade the lower respiratory tract in infants under 1 year old causing bronchiolitis or pneumonia.

Clinical features

Bronchiolitis usually starts with nasal obstruction and discharge followed by fever, cough, rapid breathing, expiratory wheezes and signs of respiratory distress such as cyanosis and inspiratory indrawing of the intercostal spaces.

Pneumonia: in respiratory syncytial virus pneumonia there is a similar clinical picture with fever, cyanosis, prostration and rapid breathing but without expiratory wheezing.
    Bronchiolitis and pneumonia are severe diseases with a mortality rate of from 2 to 5 per cent.

Immunopathology. Inactivated vaccine against this virus enhanced the incidence of bronchiolitis and pneumonia in vaccinees compared to controls; since the diseases appear mainly in infants in whom maternal antibody is still present, it seemed probable that both diseases might be at least partly *immunological*, e.g. possibly due to the formation of immune complexes. Alternatively, the susceptibility of very young infants of these diseases may be *mechanical* and caused by the narrowness of the bronchiolar lumen: when this is inflamed, serious obstruction may be produced more readily than in older infants with wider bronchioles. This second explanation is now the more widely accepted.

Common colds. Respiratory syncytial virus also causes common colds without lower respiratory tract involvement: these are seen in older children and — rarely — in adults as well as infants.

Age. Bronchiolitis and pneumonia are almost confined to infants under one year old and are most common in those aged less than 6 months; common colds due to respiratory syncytial virus are mainly seen in pre-school children.

Epidemiology. Every year there are outbreaks of respiratory syncytial virus during the later winter months especially from February to April.

Virology
1. Paramyxovirus, one serological type.
2. RNA virus.
3. Pleomorphic enveloped particles, medium size, 90 to 130 nm; helical symmetry (Fig. 5.1).
4. Grows in cells with synctial CPE.
5. Does not haemagglutinate.

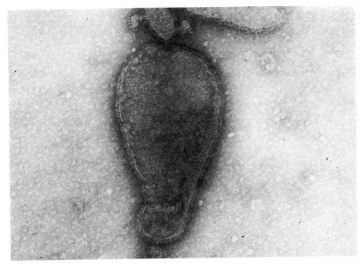

Fig. 5.1 Respiratory syncytial virus. Pleomorphic virus with helical nucleocapsid surrounded by an envelope. × 90 000. (Photograph by Dr E.A.C. Follett.)

Diagnosis

Direct demonstration of virus in respiratory secretions by immunofluorescence is now the fastest and most widely used method of diagnosis.

Isolation

Specimens: mouth washings, nasal secretions (not frozen during delivery because the virus is inactivated by freezing).

Inoculate: HeLa cells (Bristol strain), HEp-2 cells.

Observe: for characteristic CPE of syncytia of multinucleated giant cells.

Type virus: by immunofluorescence or by complement fixation test with standard antiserum.

Serology
Complement fixation test

RHINOVIRUSES

Rhinoviruses are the main cause of common colds — the most common of all infectious diseases and by far the most frequent form of respiratory infection.

Clinical features

Incubation period: 2 to 4 days.

Signs and symptoms. Nasal discharge with nasal obstruction, sneezing, sore throat and cough; about half the patients are mildly febrile; hoarseness and headache are common especially in adults.

Duration. On average symptoms subside in about a week but are prolonged for up to 2 weeks in a proportion of cases; complications are rare.

Age. Rhinovirus infections are most frequent in pre-school children; thereafter the attack rate falls but infections remain common even amongst adults.

Incidence. The reported attack rate for rhinovirus infections varies in different reports but on average the attack rate is about 0.7 rhinovirus infections per person per year.

Seasonal incidence. Infections are found all year round but the incidence is highest in autumn and winter.

Immunity. Neutralising antibody is formed after rhinovirus infection and this has a protective effect against re-infection with the particular serotype responsible.

Epidemiology. This is complex as would be expected from the large number of different virus serotypes. In any community at a given time, several serotypes can be found circulating; over a long period of time, however, there is a gradual change in the serotypes present possibly due to increasing immunity within the population to earlier serotypes.

Virology
1. Picornaviruses (pico = small + RNA); more than 100 serotypes.
2. RNA viruses.
3. Small, icosahedral particles, 20 to 30 nm.
4. Inactivated at acid pH (unlike enteroviruses — the other members of the picornavirus group).
5. Grow in tissue cultures but at 33°C, instead of the usual 37°C (the temperature of the nostrils is 33°C).
6. Two groups of viruses:
   a. 'M' rhinoviruses grow in monkey kidney tissue culture with CPE.
   b. 'H' rhinoviruses grow only in human embryo cells—with CPE: a larger group than the 'M' viruses.

Diagnosis

Isolation

Specimens: nasal secretions, mouth washings.

Inoculate: human embryo lung and monkey kidney cell cultures.

Observe: for CPE.

Type virus: by neutralisation with standard antisera.

Serology
Impractical because of the large number of serological types of rhinovirus.

Note: Laboratory diagnosis of common colds is too time-consuming for routine purposes and is therefore restricted to epidemiological research.

ADENOVIRUSES

Clinical features
Clinically, the main symptoms of adenovirus respiratory infection

are *pharyngitis and conjunctivitis*. The main syndromes are usually classified as shown in Table 5.2.

Table 5.2 Syndromes associated with adenoviruses

Syndrome	Adenovirus types
1. *Epidemic infection* pharyngo-conjunctival fever, acute respiratory disease	3, 4, 7, 14, 21
2. *Endemic infection* pharyngitis, follicular conjunctivitis	1 2, 3, 5, 6, 7
3. *Epidemic kerato-conjunctivitis or 'shipyard eye'*	8

1. *Epidemic infection*: common in recruit camps where attack rates of 70 per cent have been reported; also seen in children's institutions due to crowding together of susceptible young hosts.
2. *Endemic infection*: adenovirus infections are endemic but at a low level in the general population: they usually constitute less than 5 per cent of the respiratory infections in the community at large; types 1, 2, 5 and 6 are associated with endemic infection, but cases of infection due to types 3 and 7 are common in the community and tend to be found in clusters.
3. *Epidemic kerato-conjunctivitis*: a form of eye infection which is spread mainly by contaminated instruments at eye clinics and surgeries; epidemics are seen in eye patients and also in shipyard and metal workers who are prone to minor eye injuries which require treatment at eye clinics: unlike the other forms of adenovirus disease, this disease is usually associated with only one adenovirus — type 8.

Alimentary tract
Adenoviruses are common in the alimentary as well as the respiratory tract; this is probably due to their predilection for lymphoid tissue; adenoviruses may play a role in mesenteric adenitis and intussusception in children.

Oncogenic properties
Several adenoviruses cause cancer on injection into hamsters; the most highly oncogenic are types 12, 18 and 31. However, adenoviruses do not cause tumours in man.

Chronic infection
Adenoviruses have a tendency to persist for long periods in tissues such as the tonsils and adenoids: this may not be true latency but rather a low grade persistent infectious process.

Virology

1. 33 serological types which react independently in neutralisation tests; but all adenoviruses share a common group complement-fixing antigen.
2. DNA viruses.
3. Medium size: 60 to 70 nm; icosahedron-shaped particles with cubic symmetry and with fibres topped with knobs projecting from the vertices (Fig. 5.2).
4. Most haemagglutinate.
5. Grow slowly in tissue cultures, (human embryonic cells or HeLa cells are best) with CPE of clusters of rounded and 'ballooned' cells.

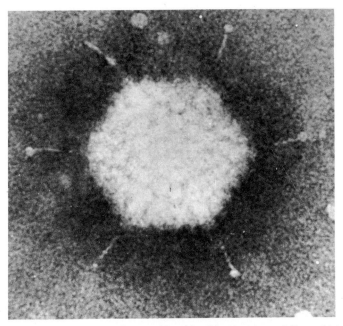

Fig. 5.2 Adenovirus. Icosahedron particle with cubic symmetry and fibres which project from the vertices. × 200 000. (Reproduced, with permission, from Valentine, R.C. & Pereira, H.G., 1965, *Journal of Molecular Biology*, **13**, 13)

DIAGNOSIS

Isolation

Specimens: mouth washings, throat swabs, faeces.

Inoculate: human embryonic cell cultures or HeLa cells.

Observe: for characteristic CPE of large rounded cells arranged like 'bunches of grapes'.

Type virus by neutralisation test.

Serology

Complement fixation test. Adenoviruses share a common group complement-fixing antigen (although they differ antigenically in neutralisation tests).

By testing patients' sera against adenovirus group antigen in complement fixation tests, adenovirus infection can be diagnosed, but this gives no indication of the serotype of the adenovirus responsible.

OTHER VIRUSES CAUSING COMMON COLDS

Coronaviruses

Medium sized (80 to 100 nm) RNA viruses; the virus particles are unusual and resemble those of avian bronchitis and mouse hepatitis; the spherical enveloped particles are surrounded by a fringe of club-shaped projections; isolated in organ cultures of human embryo trachea where virus may be detected by ciliary immobilisation or by electron microscopy of the culture; some strains can be adapted to growth in the L132 line of human embryo lung cells with CPE. There are at least 3 antigenic types although with some antigenic cross-reactions or sharing between the types.

Coronaviruses are probably common causes of colds in the community but the difficulty of isolating them in the laboratory means that they are seldom diagnosed.

Enteroviruses

Some enteroviruses cause respiratory infections; the main types associated with respiratory disease are Coxsackievirus A21 (Coe virus), B3 and echovirus types 11 and 20.

6

Neurological disease due to viruses

Neurological disease is a serious and not uncommon complication of virus infection. Most human pathogenic viruses are capable of spreading to the central nervous system (CNS).

Virus lesions in the CNS are due mainly to *viral multiplication* in the cells of the nervous tissues with cellular damage and dysfunction and consequent neurological signs and symptoms. But the *immune response of the host* may also play a role in causing lesions. Lesions may be due to an antigen-antibody reaction in the tissues — with resulting inflammatory response — rather than to virus multiplication alone. In one form of viral CNS disease (post-infectious encephalomyelitis) virus cannot be isolated from the CNS.

Spread: most viruses invade the CNS *by the blood stream* but some, e.g. rabies, reach the CNS by the *neural route* as a result of spreading along the peripheral nerves.
 CNS involvement is not always followed by neurological disease — for example there is evidence that *symptomless involvement of the CNS* is common in measles and mumps.

 Virus neurological diseases fall into two clinical categories — acute and chronic.

ACUTE VIRAL NEUROLOGICAL DISEASE:

There are four main syndromes:
1. *Encephalitis.* The main symptoms are drowsiness, mental confusion, convulsions, focal neurological signs and sometimes coma.
2. *Paralysis.* With fever, flaccid paralysis — most often of the lower limbs — and signs of meningitis such as headache with stiffness of neck and back.

Table 6.1 Acute virus neurological diseases

	Direct invasion of CNS by virus			Virus not demonstrable in CNS (disease is probably due to abnormal immune response of host to infection)
Disease	Encephalitis		Paralysis (anterior poliomyelitis)	Aseptic meningitis	Post-infectious encephalomyelitis.
Site	Brain		Anterior horn cells of spinal cord	Meninges	Brain
Lesions	Destructive lesions in grey matter; neuronal damage		Destructive lesions of lower motor neurones with meningitis	Inflammation of meninges, cells in CSF (usually lymphocytes)	Perivascular infiltration, microglial proliferation, demyelination
Viruses	Herpes simplex, togaviruses, rabies		Enteroviruses (especially polioviruses)	Enteroviruses, mumps, lymphocytic chorio-meningitis	Measles, rubella, varicella-zoster vaccinia

Table 6.2 Chronic virus neurological diseases

Disease	Subacute sclerosing panencephalitis	Progressive multifocal leucoencephalopathy	Kuru	Creutzfeldt-Jakob disease
Site	Brain	Brain	Brain	Brain and spinal cord
Lesions	Neuronal degeneration, intranuclear inclusions	Multiple foci of degeneration	Spongiform degeneration especially in cerebellum	Spongiform degeneration
Viruses	Measles, rubella (after congenital infection)	JC virus, human SV$_{40}$-like virus	Transmissible by filter-passing agent	Transmissible by filter-passing agent

3. *Aseptic meningitis*. A relatively mild disease with fever, headache and stiffness of neck and back.
4. *Post-infectious encephalomyelitis* (also called encephalitis). Symptoms are similar to those of encephalitis.

Table 6.1 summarises the principal features of the four main acute viral neurological syndromes.

CHRONIC VIRUS NEUROLOGICAL DISEASES

Viruses cause several chronic neurological diseases which are listed in Table 6.2. The diseases are described in more detail in the chapters on the viruses which cause them but below are some of the main features:

1. *Rare*. All the diseases are very rare and most doctors will probably never see a case of any of them throughout their working lives.
2. *Signs and symptoms*. Numerous and varied but are neurological and often affect intellectual capacity as well as both motor and sensory functions.
3. *Duration*. The diseases may last for months or even years but are relentlessly progressive.
4. *Fatal*. The diseases are always fatal.

7

Enterovirus infections; infantile gastroenteritis

Enteroviruses are a large family of viruses, of which the main site of infection is the gut; however, they rarely cause intestinal symptoms; enterovirus diseases are the result of spread of the viruses to other sites in the body — particularly the CNS.

Below are listed the various groups included in the enterovirus family:

Enteroviruses

	polioviruses	Coxsackieviruses*		echoviruses**	enteroviruses (unclassified)
		group A	group B		
types	1–3	1–24	1–6	1–34	68–71

*Coxsackie is the village in New York where these viruses were first isolated.
**Enteric, Cytopathic, Human, Orphan (because originally — but wrongly — thought not to be associated with human disease).

Enteroviruses have the following properties:

Enter the body via ingestion by mouth.

Primary site of multiplication is the lymphoid tissue of the alimentary tract — including the pharynx.

Spread from the gut is in two directions:
1. *Outwards* into the blood (viraemia) and so to other tissues and organs.
2. *Inwards* into the lumen of the gut and to excretion in the faeces.

Clinical features

Note: Enteroviruses do not cause gastroenteritis.

The main enterovirus diseases are shown in Table 7.1.

Table 7.1 Enterovirus diseases

Syndrome	Main viruses responsible
1. Neurological	
(i) Paralysis	polioviruses
(ii) Aseptic meningitis	most enteroviruses
2. Febrile illness	most enteroviruses
3. Herpangina; hand, foot and mouth disease	Coxsackie A viruses
4. Myocarditis; pericarditis	Coxsackie B viruses
5. Bornholm disease	Coxsackie B viruses
6. Acute haemorrhagic conjunctivitis	enterovirus 70

General features of enterovirus infections
Most enterovirus infections are confined to the alimentary tract and are symptomless.

A *small proportion* of infections give rise to febrile illness due to viraemia.

A *few cases* progress to aseptic meningitis but spread of virus to the CNS or other organs and tissues is a rare complication of enterovirus infection.

NEUROLOGICAL SYNDROMES

Neurological disease is the most important manifestation of enteroviral infection; it is not associated with one particular group or type of enterovirus.

The illness is usually biphasic: the initial symptoms are of a febrile illness due to viraemia; there is an intervening period of well-being for a day or two followed by the onset of neurological symptoms; these are due to spread of the virus through the 'blood-brain barrier' to invade the CNS.

There are two main types of neurological disease due to enteroviruses:
1. *Paralysis* or poliomyelitis: an acute illness with pain and *flaccid* paralysis affecting mainly the lower legs. Sometimes the muscles of respiration become involved requiring tracheostomy with con-

trolled breathing by positive-pressure respirator; more rarely, the disease may take the form of *bulbar paralysis* when the muscles of breathing and swallowing are primarily involved. Paralysis is associated with the signs and symptoms of aseptic meningitis.

Pathology: paralysis is due to viral damage to the cells of the anterior horn of the spinal cord: this causes lower motor neurone lesions resulting in flaccid paralysis. If damage to the nerve cells is severe, the paralysis may be permanent.

Paralysis is most often due to the three polioviruses and especially poliovirus 1. Before the introduction of poliovaccine, epidemics of paralysis were common in countries with a high standard of living e.g. USA, Denmark and Australia.

2. *Aseptic meningitis*: signs of neurological disease are present but the damage is minor and there is no paralysis; the main signs and symptoms are fever and headache with nuchal rigidity (stiffness of the neck muscles due to meningeal irritation). Lymphocytes and protein in the cerebrospinal fluid (CSF) are increased. The prognosis is good and most patients recover completely — although some minor neurological sequelae have been found in cases followed up after discharge from hospital.

Epidemics of aseptic meningitis are common: these are often due to echovirus 9 or, before widespread use of poliovaccine, to polioviruses; echoviruses 4, 6 and 30 and Coxsackieviruses A7, A9 and B5 are also sometimes associated with epidemic aseptic meningitis.

NON–NEUROLOGICAL SYNDROMES

Enterovirus infection which proceeds to viraemia commonly presents as an acute, although usually mild, febrile illness. Some enteroviruses, notably Coxsackie A16 and echovirus 9 regularly cause a rash which accompanies the fever.

Some non-neurological syndromes associated with a particular enterovirus group are listed below:

Herpangina: a painful eruption of vesicles in the mouth and throat: recently, it has been reported as part of the syndrome of 'hand, foot and mouth disease' in which there are vesicles also on the hands and feet; due to group A Coxsackieviruses; enterovirus 71 has also caused hand, foot and mouth disease.

Bornholm disease: also known as pleurodynia or epidemic myalgia: a painful inflammation of muscles which mainly involves the inter-costal muscles. The disease is named after the Danish island where there was an extensive outbreak in 1930; due to group B Coxsack-ieviruses.

Myocarditis and pericarditis: due to Group B Coxsackieviruses. *Myocarditis* is characterized by rapid pulse, enlargement of the heart and ECG abnormalities and *pericarditis* by pericardial friction or effusion.

Each syndrome can be present on its own but patients often de-velop myocarditis and pericarditis together. Both diseases are seen mainly in adult males, and may be mistaken for myocardial infarc-tion; however, the prognosis is good and most patients recover completely. Rarely epidemics have been reported among neonates in hospital nurseries. In the 1965 epidemic of Coxsackievirus B5 in-fections in England and Wales, 5% of the patients had cardiac signs or symptoms the incidence being higher in adults than in children.

Acute haemorrhagic conjunctivitis: due to enterovirus 70 has ap-peared in large-scale outbreaks in 1969–71 in Africa, South East Asia, Japan, India and to a limited extent in Britain. There is an in-cubation period of 24 hours and the disease spreads rapidly, prob-ably via eye discharges; the disease lasts about 10 days and patients recover completely. Unlike most enterovirus infections the causal virus is not found in the faeces.

Epidemiology

Enterovirus infections are common — especially in children and in conditions of poor hygiene.

Infection is spread mainly by the faecal-oral route from virus excre-tors to contacts; virus in pharyngeal secretions may also be a source of infection.

Gut immunity: after infection with an enterovirus, the gut becomes resistant to reinfection with the same enterovirus; this resistance is due to the production in the gut of virus-specific neutralising IgA antibody.

Seasonal distribution: infections are far more frequent in the sum-mer than in the winter months.

Predominant strains: one or two enterovirus types usually predominate in a season; the types which emerge are determined by the level of immunity in the population concerned; this in turn depends on the previous infections experienced by the community.

Poor sanitation, e.g. in under-developed countries, increases the chances of childhood infection so that immunity is acquired early in life.

High standard of living in countries such as the USA, diminishes the chance of infection and therefore of immunity being acquired in childhood.

Adults are more liable to develop severe paralysis in poliovirus infection than children: the risk of this is increased by pregnancy, tonsillectomy, fatigue, trauma or inoculation with bacterial vaccines.

Epidemics: countries with a high standard of living have a relatively large proportion of non-immune adults and before the advent of poliovaccines suffered from repeated and widespread epidemics of paralytic disease.

Virology
1. Picornaviruses (pico = small + RNA): numerous serological types.
2. RNA viruses.
3. Small roughly spherical particles, 25 to 30 nm (Fig. 7.1).
4. Stable at acid pH (in contrast to the rhinoviruses — the other members of the picornavirus group).
5. Most grow in tissue cultures with rapid production of CPE.
6. Coxsackieviruses (but not polio or echoviruses) are pathogenic for suckling mice.

Diagnosis

Isolation

Specimens: faeces, throat swabs: CSF is useful for some viruses (e.g. echovirus 9) but not for polioviruses.

Inoculate: monkey kidney, human embryo lung or RD cell cultures.

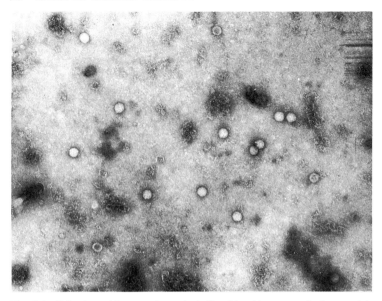

Fig. 7.1 Echovirus. All enteroviruses look like this with very small virus particles with cubic symmetry. × 90 000. (Photograph by Dr E.A.C. Follett.)

Observe: for CPE.

Type virus: by neutralisation tests with standard antisera; usually done using pooled antisera to reduce the number of tests.

Note: Most Coxsackie A viruses do not grow in tissue cultures so if Coxsackie A virus infection is suspected:

Inoculate: suckling mice subcutaneously and intracerebrally.

Observe: for characteristic signs of disease.
   Group A Coxsackieviruses cause flaccid paralysis due to widespread myositis.
   Group B Coxsackieviruses cause spastic paralysis with tremor due to cerebral lesions and fat-pad necrosis.

Serology

Coxsackie B virus infection. Neutralisation tests are useful for the diagnosis of Coxsackie B virus infections, e.g. myocarditis, pericarditis, Bornholm disease.

Apart from this, the large number of enteroviruses make serological diagnosis impracticable.

Vaccination
Two vaccines were originally produced against the most paralytogenic enteroviruses, i.e. the three polioviruses.

1. *Sabin live attenuated virus vaccine*
Now the main vaccine used for poliomyelitis immunisation.

Contains the three polioviruses as attenuated strains which have lost neurovirulence for monkeys (i.e. ability to produce paralysis or lesions in CNS of monkeys); grown in monkey kidney tissue cultures.

Administered in three oral doses along with triple vaccine starting at 6 months of age.

Protection: good.

Blood antibody response: good.

Gut immunity: good, vaccinated children show increased resistance to alimentary infection; this is due to the appearance of virus-specific IgA in the gut produced in response to the vaccine.

Safety: good; very rarely paralysis — usually mild and usually due to the type 3 component: incidence about 1 per million doses.

Vaccinated children are infectious to others so that vaccine strains may circulate to some extent in the community.

Widespread use of this vaccine has resulted in a dramatic decrease both in paralytic poliomyelitis and in the circulation of wild polioviruses in the community.

2. *Salk inactivated virus vaccine*
This was the first polio vaccine to be used on a large scale but has now been largely replaced by Sabin vaccine. It contains the three polioviruses inactivated by formaldehyde and is given in three injections. Although producing good blood antibody levels — and therefore good protection against paralysis — it fails to give gut immunity.

INFANTILE GASTROENTERITIS

Also known as acute non-bacterial gastroenteritis, this disease causes acute diarrhoea in infants; in Britain today the disease is generally mild but is an important cause of infant mortality in under-developed countries. Several viruses are implicated but the main cause of the disease is rotavirus. Rotavirus is a genus within the reovirus family (i.e. viruses with a fragmented double-stranded RNA genome and a double layered capsid).

Clinical features

Incubation period: 1 to 4 days.

Symptoms: Acute onset of vomiting — which is sometimes projectile — and diarrhoea; dehydration is common and may require intravenous fluid replacement as a life-saving emergency procedure: respiratory symptoms e.g. cough, coryza, are common.

Duration: About a week.

Age: Most common in infants — i.e. under 2 years old — and especially in babies less than one year old; although rarer, cases have been reported in adults.

Epidemics are common especially amongst babies in nurseries.

Seasonal: infections are more common in winter than summer.

Virus is excreted in faeces — in considerable quantity — during the acute stage of illness.

Virology
1. Virus particles, 65 nm diameter with a characteristic wheel-like appearance of their two-layered capsid (Fig. 7.2).
2. Two serological types.
3. Does not grow in tissue culture.
4. Morphologically identical and antigenically related to the virus of calf diarrhoea.

Diagnosis

Demonstration of virus by:
1. Electron microscopy to detect typical virus particles in faecal samples.

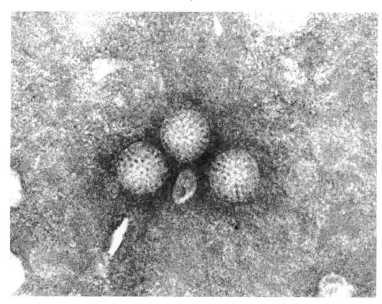

Fig. 7.2 Rotavirus. Spherical particles with cubic symmetry, showing characteristic outer layer like the spokes of a wheel which distinguishes the virus from reovirus. × 200 000. (Photograph by Prof. C.R. Madeley.)

2. Serological tests for virus antigen in faeces by complement fixation or EIA tests.

Other viruses causing gastroenteritis
Caliciviruses, astroviruses and 'small round viruses' (i.e. undifferentiated small virus particles) have been seen in the stool of patients with acute infantile gastroenteritis: their significance in the disease is uncertain: none of the viruses grows in tissue culture.

Winter vomiting disease is a syndrome of acute vomiting but variable diarrhoea in which the symptoms overlap with those of acute gastroenteritis: there is evidence that many cases are associated with caliciviruses (picorna-like viruses found in many animal species as well as man).

8

Arthropod-borne virus infections

Many important virus diseases are transmitted by the bite of an arthropod vector. The viruses are therefore called *arboviruses*; these include many unrelated viruses belonging to different families.

Togaviruses
The largest family of arboviruses, they are subdivided into alphaviruses (formerly group A arboviruses) and flaviviruses (formerly group B arboviruses). Togaviruses multiply in the bodies of arthropod vectors without producing disease and may be excreted from them for months after infection.

Other arboviruses
Bunyaviruses (enveloped RNA viruses larger than togaviruses with helical symmetry and a fragmented genome) and orbiviruses (a genus within the reovirus family).

Vectors: Mosquitoes, ticks and sandflies are the principal arthropod vectors which transmit arboviruses.

Animal hosts. The main reservoirs are wild birds and small mammals; the viruses spread to man when an arthropod vector acquires virus from its natural host and transmits it by biting the human host.

Disease. Arboviruses cause two main types of disease:
1. Encephalitis
2. Fever (sometimes with haemorrhage)
   Some of the most important arboviruses are listed in Table 8.1 together with their vectors and the diseases they produce.

ARBOVIRUS ENCEPHALITIS

Arbovirus encephalitis is a world-wide problem. It is common in America (Eastern, Western and Venezuelan equine encephalitis,

Table 8.1 Classification of arboviruses

Virus	Disease	Vector
Alphaviruses		
Eastern equine encephalitis	Encephalitis	Mosquito
Western equine encephalitis	Encephalitis	Mosquito
Venezuelan equine encephalitis	Encephalitis, febrile disease	Mosquito
O'nyong-nyong	Febrile disease	Mosquito
Chikungunya	Febrile disease, haemorrhagic fever	Mosquito
Flaviviruses		
St Louis encephalitis	Encephalitis	Mosquito
Japanese B encephalitis	Encephalitis	Mosquito
Murray Valley encephalitis	Encephalitis	Mosquito
Tick-borne encephalitis	Encephalitis	Tick
Yellow fever	Haemorrhagic fever	Mosquito
Kyasanur Forest fever	Haemorrhagic fever	Tick
Dengue	Febrile disease, haemorrhagic fever	Mosquito
Bunyaviruses		
California encephalitis	Encephalitis	Mosquito
Rift Valley fever	Febrile disease, haemorrhagic fever	Mosquito
Congo/Crimean haemorrhagic fever	Haemorrhagic fever	Tick
Orbivirus		
Colorado tick fever	Febrile disease	Tick

California and St Louis encephalitis), the Far East (Japanese B encephalitis), Eastern Europe (tick-borne encephalitis) and Australia (Murray Valley encephalitis). It is not a problem in Britain where the only arbovirus found is that causing the tick-borne disease, louping ill, in sheep.

Clinically, the main symptoms are fever, progressively severe headache, nausea, vomiting, stiffness of neck, back and legs; there may be convulsions, drowsiness, deepening coma or neurological signs such as paralysis and tremor.

Symptomless infection is common with most of the arboviruses which cause encephalitis. After an epidemic, arbovirus antibodies are often present in a considerable proportion of the population; the incidence of encephalitis with arbovirus infection is usually low although some viruses, e.g. Eastern equine encephalitis virus, cause symptoms in a much higher proportion of people infected than others, e.g. the viruses of Western equine and St Louis encephalitis. Eastern equine encephalitis also has a higher mortality rate.

Age. Arbovirus encephalitis affects all ages although some variations are seen with different viruses. For example, California encephalitis is mainly seen in school children whereas St Louis encephalitis produces its most severe effects in older people in whom neurological sequelae are common; Western equine encephalitis on the other hand is more severe in young people.

Epidemics of arbovirus encephalitis are common and have been well studied in the USA: epidemics are seasonal, infection being more frequent in summer and autumn. Before and during a human epidemic there is evidence of infection spreading in the animals, e.g. birds, that are the natural hosts of the virus; in Eastern, Western and Venezuelan equine encephalitis, epidemics of human infection are preceded by or concurrent with epidemic infection in horses. The horses, like man, are secondary hosts of the viruses, the primary or natural hosts being birds (Eastern and Western) and small mammals (Venezuelan).

ARBOVIRUS FEVERS AND HAEMORRHAGIC FEVERS

These syndromes overlap to some extent in that haemorrhages are not infrequent complications of arbovirus fevers; there is some evidence that the haemorrhagic forms of disease may be due to formation of immune complexes due to abnormally large production of antibodies.

Note: haemorrhagic fevers are also caused by other, non-arthropod-borne viruses (see p. 74).

Epidemiology. Worldwide in distribution especially in semi-tropical and tropical countries; epidemics are frequent and are a major health problem. Symptomless infection — detected by a relatively high incidence of antibodies in the general population concerned — is common.

Clinically, the symptoms are those of a severe generalized febrile disease with high fever, chills, severe headache, pain in the limbs, nausea and vomiting; some arbovirus fevers have additional and characteristic signs and symptoms.

Below are some of the best known arbovirus fevers:

Yellow fever
Endemic in South America and the central belt of Africa. There are two forms:
1. *Urban* in which the reservoir of the virus is man and the vector the mosquito *Aedes aegypti*.
2. *Sylvan or jungle* in which the reservoir is tree-dwelling monkeys and the vector various species of forest mosquito.

Clinically, the most striking feature of yellow fever is jaundice due to viral invasion of the liver causing hepatitis; haemorrhages are often seen and a toxic nephrosis with proteinuria is a common feature.

Kyasanur Forest fever
A haemorrhagic fever seen mainly in forest workers in Mysore State, India: the animal reservoirs are monkeys and possibly small mammals also.

Dengue
Dengue is a major health problem in South-east Asia, India, the Pacific Islands, and the Caribbean; infection is widespread in these areas; monkeys are probably the main reservoir of infection and the main vector is *Aedes aegypti*.

Antigenic types: there are four sub-types (types 1 to 4) of dengue virus.

Clinically, dengue typically presents the classical features of a severe febrile disease with pain in the limbs and rash; the case fatality rate of this type of dengue is low.

Dengue haemorrhagic shock syndrome is a serious complication of dengue seen in young children. In this syndrome, an attack of dengue progresses to a more severe disease characterized by haemorrhages and the symptoms of shock; this form is apparently seen in children who have experienced a previous attack of dengue due to a different sub-type of virus: on re-infection with a second sub-type of virus, immune complexes are formed due to production of excess antibody following the first attack which reacts with the second virus; the immune complexes are responsible for the haemorrhagic shock syndrome.

Chikunguna and O'nyong-nyong

The cause of widespread epidemics of febrile disease in Africa.

Clinically, both diseases are characterized by severe pain in the joints: O'nyong-nyong is a dialect name meaning break-bone fever. Residual joint pains may persist after recovery from the acute disease.

Haemorrhagic fever: both diseases sometimes cause haemorrhagic fever and, occasionally, shock syndromes.

Rift Valley fever

Responsible for large epizootics in sheep and cattle in Africa – particularly Egypt, the Sudan and South Africa. Human infection is acquired through contact with infected animals. The human disease is a febrile disease with haemorrhages in severe cases: some patients have developed retinitis.

Congo/ Crimean haemorrhagic fever

This is seen in Southern Russia, Bulgaria and in West and East Africa: more recently the disease has been reported in the Middle East and Pakistan.

Clinically, the disease has a high mortality rate: the most serious cases show a marked haemorrhagic tendency sometimes with extensive skin ecchymoses. There is evidence that severely haemorrhagic cases have a greater antibody response than patients with milder disease.

Virology

The following are the main properties of togaviruses:
1. More than 300 serological types.
2. RNA viruses.
3. Roughly spherical, enveloped particles most are between 40 and 70 nm (Fig. 8.1).
4. Most haemagglutinate avian erythrocyctes, e.g. from day-old chicks or geese.
5. Pathogenic for suckling mice.
6. Grow in tissue culture.

Note: rubella virus is now classified as a togavirus: it is not arthropod-borne and, since it causes a different disease from that asso-

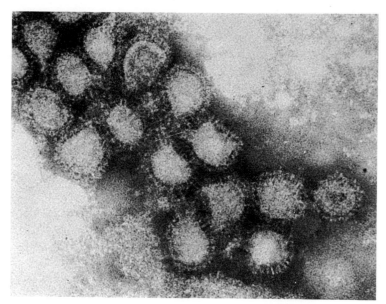

Fig 8.1 Togavirus. This photograph of sindbis virus shows roughly spherical particles with cubic symmetry and a surface fringe. × 200 000. (Photograph by Prof. C.R. Madeley.)

ciated with other togaviruses, it is described separately in Chapter 11.

Diagnosis

Serology
Complement fixation tests.
Haemagglutination-inhibition tests (of limited value).
Neutralisation.

Isolation (difficult)

Specimens: blood, throat swab, CSF.

Inoculate: suckling mice intra-cerebrally.

Observe: for up to 15 days for tremors, failure to eat, wasting, paralysis.

On death: Harvest brain and liver.

Type: Identify by haemagglutination-inhibition and complement fixation test.

Yellow fever vaccine

Contains live attenuated virus of a strain known as 17D attenuated by repeated passage in chick embryos.

Prepared in chick embryos

Administered in one dose by subcutaneous injection.

Protection conferred is good, solid immunity which lasts for at least 10 years.

Safety: good, singularly free from side-effects.

9

Rabies, Marburg disease, arenavirus infections

RABIES

Rabies is a lethal form of encephalitis due to a virus which affects a wide variety of animal species: rabies is transmitted to man via the bite of an infected animal which is usually — but not always — a dog.

Clinical features

The incubation period is long — usually from 4 to 12 weeks but sometimes much longer; if the wound is on the head or neck the incubation period is shorter than for wounds on the limbs.

Virus spread from the wound to the CNS is via the nerves.

Symptoms: mainly of excitement, with tremor, muscular contractions and convulsions; typically spasm of the muscles of swallowing (hence the older name for the disease of 'hydrophobia' or fear of water) and increased sensitivity of the sensory nervous system. Virus is present in saliva, skin and eyes.

Prognosis: the disease is virtually always fatal; death often follows a convulsion.

Pathology: despite the severity of the clinical disease, lesions in the CNS are often minimal with little evidence of destructive effect on cells; the main changes are the typical intracytoplasmic inclusions within neurones known as Negri bodies.

Another type of rabies is seen in the West Indies, and Central and South America: this takes the form of *ascending myelitis with paralysis* and lesions are found in the ganglion cells of the spinal cord; it is spread by the bite of infected vampire bats.

Epidemiology

Rabies is a natural infection of dogs, cats, bats and carnivorous wild animals such as foxes, wolves, skunks and, sometimes, cattle. At present, rabies is generally more common in cats than dogs — except in Turkey where dog rabies is a particular problem.

Virus is present in the saliva of infected animals — sometimes for up to four days before the onset of symptoms of the disease; animals which remain healthy for ten days after biting can be regarded as being free of virus at the time of biting.

Incidence of rabies after biting: relatively few — possibly only about 15% — of people bitten by a rabid animal develop the disease; rabies is more common after bites on the head or neck than after wounds on the limbs.

Britain is at present free from indigenous rabies. Rabies used to be present in animals in Britain but was eradicated by 1921; the strict six month-quarantine laws for animals imported into Britain have on the whole been successful in keeping out the disease. Smuggling of pet animals into Britain to avoid the quarantine regulations is fairly common and represents a potential source of importation of the virus. The main danger is that rabies might become established as a reservoir of infection in wild animals. If this happens, it would be extremely difficult to eradicate the disease. Rabies is present in wild animals in Europe, USA and most other areas of the world and, most important from a British point of view, in the area on the French side of the English Channel.

Corneal transplant: cases of rabies in recipients of corneas from donors with undiagnosed rabies have been reported.

Virology

1. Rhabdovirus: one serological type.
2. RNA virus.
3. Bullet-shaped, enveloped particles containing helically-coiled nucleo-protein; length 180 nm, diameter 70 to 80 nm (Fig. 9.1).
4. Haemagglutinates goose erythrocytes.
5. Grows in hamster kidney and chick embryo cell tissue cultures with eosinophilic cytoplasmic inclusions but usually without CPE.
6. Pathogenic for mice and other laboratory animals.

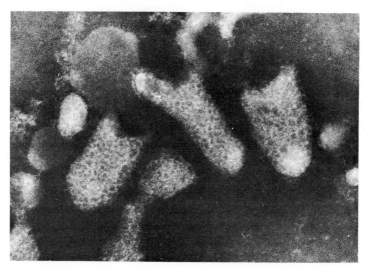

Fig. 9.1 Rabies virus. The nucleocapsid of the bullet-shaped particles has helical symmetry and is surrounded by an envelope. × 180 000. (Photograph by Prof. C.R. Madeley.)

Diagnosis

Direct demonstration of virus

Specimens: hair-bearing skin (e.g. back of neck), corneal impression smears, brain tissue.

Examine: for presence of rabies viral antigen by immunofluorescence.

Negri bodies: a less sensitive method of diagnosis: examine brain smears of the Ammon's horn of the hippocampus stained with Seller's stain for red intracytoplasmic inclusions (Negri bodies.)

Isolation

Specimens: brain tissue, saliva, CSF, urine.

Inoculate: mice intra-cerebrally.

Observe: for paralysis, convulsions; *post-mortem* for immunofluorescence with rabies antiserum and Negri bodies in brain cells. **Note**: If rabies is suspected in a dog it should be kept under observation to see if the disease develops, and not killed right away; if it is killed before death due to the disease, Negri bodies may not have developed in sufficient numbers to be detected in histological sections.

Vaccination

Rabies vaccine was first developed by Pasteur in 1885; it consisted of virus attenuated by drying the spinal cords of infected rabbits for varying lenghts of time over KOH. Wild rabies virus is known as 'street' virus and attenuated virus as 'fixed' virus. All vaccines prepared for human use contain inactivated virus.

The long incubation period makes rabies a suitable disease for prophylactic immunisation after exposure.

After exposure — or suspicion of exposure — to rabies, the wound should be thoroughly washed with soap and water, alcohol, iodine solutions or quarternary ammonium compound; patients should then be given combined passive and active immunisation.

Passive immunisation: injection of human anti-rabies immunoglobulin.

Active immunisation: should be started after passive immunisation. The main vaccines in use are :

1. **Human diploid cell vaccine** — now the vaccine of choice.
   Contains: inactivated virus disrupted into subunits.
   Prepared: in WI 38 human embryo lung cells.
   Administered: intramuscularly or subcutaneously in 6 doses spaced at 0, 3, 7, 14, 30 and 90 days.
   Protection: apparently effective; produces high levels of neutralizing antibody.
   Safety: Good: does not cause neuroparalytic complications.

2. **Duck embryo killed virus vaccine**
   Contains: inactivated virus.
   Prepared: in duck embryos; although a crude tissue emulsion, it contains very little nervous tissue.
   Administered: subcutaneously in 14–21 daily injections with later booster doses.
   Protection: apparently effective although slightly less potent than brain tissue vaccine.
   Safety: good.

3. **Semple vaccine**
   Contains: virus inactivated by phenol.
   Prepared: from virus in infected rabbit brain tissue.
   Administered: subcutaneously in 21 daily injections with later booster doses
   Protection: apparently effective.
   Safety: neuroparalytic accidents due to allergic encephalomyeli-

tis sometimes follow immunisation as a result of the repeated injections of nervous tissue.
4. **Animal vaccines:** modified live vaccines.
   Contain: live attenuated virus — HEP (high egg passage) Flury strain, SAD (Street Alabama Dufferin strain) or Kissling strain.
   Used: for immunization of dogs, cats, cattle, etc.
Pre-exposure vaccination
Veterinary surgeons, animal handlers, laboratory workers or others at high risk from rabies should be given three doses of diploid cell vaccine one month apart with a booster dose 2 years later; two booster doses should be given if they are exposed to infection.

MARBURG VIRUS DISEASE

A severe disease popularly — but unfortunately — known as 'green monkey disease' appeared in 1967 as a single outbreak initially involving laboratory workers in Marburg, Frankfurt and Belgrade. The patients had handled tissues from the same batch of African green monkeys. Later, there were other cases in contacts of the patients. The disease apparently originated in the monkeys which were infected with the virus.

Clinical features
Clinically, the disease is a severe, febrile illness with headache, myalgia, a maculo-papular rash and haemorrhagic manifestations; other features are vomiting, diarrhoea, hepatitis and signs of renal and CNS involvement. There is leucopenia with atypical lymphocytes and plasma cells in the blood; the mortality rate was 23 % in the original outbreak.

Epidemiology
Marburg disease appeared again in 1975 in two young people in South Africa; in 1976 there were severe outbreaks with many deaths in Sudan and Zaire. These outbreaks were due to a morphologically similar but antigenically different virus now named Ebola virus.

Primates, i.e. monkeys (Marburg virus) and baboons (Ebola virus), may be the natural hosts of the viruses since antibodies have been found in a small proportion of these animals. However, in the original 1967 outbreak, the monkeys which spread the disease probably became infected in transit — possibly during a stopover in London airport.

Virology

1. Provisionally classified as a rhabdovirus.
2. RNA virus.
3. Very unusual virus particles, long, filamentous, with the ends bent forming a hook or a horseshoe shape; 665 nm by 100 nm.
4. Grows in various tissue cultures without CPE but with intracytoplasmic inclusions resembling Negri bodies.
5. Pathogenic for guinea-pigs, monkeys and other laboratory animals.

Diagnosis

The disease has a very characteristic clinical picture. Confirmation of the virus aetiology in the original outbreak was obtained by isolating the virus in laboratory animals.

Isolation

Specimen: blood.

Inoculate: guinea-pigs.

Observe: for signs of febrile illness.

Serology

Complement fixation test.

ARENAVIRUSES

LYMPHOCYTIC CHORIOMENINGITIS

Another disease contracted by man from animals. The virus causes widespread natural infection in mice and is excreted in the urine and faeces of infected mice; transmission to man appears to be a rare event.

The disease is of interest from an immunological point of view since mice are not uncommonly infected *in utero*; when this happens they have a generalised infection with high titres of virus in all tissues and organs; however the mice remain symptomless although they later succumb to glomerulonephritis due to immune complex deposition in kidneys.

Clinical features

The most important syndrome in man is aseptic meningitis; sometimes meningo-encephalitis is seen; the virus can also cause an influenza-like febrile illness.

Virus is spread to man by inhalation of dust or by contamination of food in infested houses. The disease has been acquired from pet and laboratory hamsters.

Virology
1. Arenavirus.
2. RNA virus.
3. Medium-sized virus — 110 nm enveloped particles with internal granules (which seem to be ribosomes) characteristic of arenaviruses.
4. Grows in the chick embryo and in monkey kidney and chick embryo cell tissue cultures.
5. Pathogenic for mice and guinea-pigs.

Diagnosis

Serology
Complement fixation test.

Isolation

Specimen: CSF, blood.

Inoculate: mice intra-cerebrally.

Observe: for spasm of hind legs, tremors, convulsions and death.

LASSA FEVER

A serious febrile disease endemic in West Africa which was first reported in Lassa in Nigeria. The virus is highly infectious and spreads readily by contact — including to medical and nursing personnel looking after patients. Rats are the reservoir of the virus.

Clinical features
The illness is severe with fever, vomiting, cough, weakness and malaise; sore throat with ulcers in the mouth and pharynx and cervical lymphadenopathy are characteristic features; abdominal pain, myalgia with diarrhoea and headache are common and the blood count shows leucopenia; the case fatality rate is difficult to estimate in the small outbreaks described but several patients have died.

Virology

1. Arenavirus.
2. RNA virus.
3. Medium-sized virus, enveloped particles, 110 nm in diameter, with internal granules which appear to be ribosomes derived from the host cell.
4. Grows in tissue culture — in Vero cells (a monkey kidney cell line) with CPE.
5. Non-pathogenic for mice.
6. Slight antigenic relationship with lymphocytic choriomeningitis virus.

Diagnosis

Isolation

Specimens: blood, throat washings, urine, pleural fluid.

Inoculate: Vero monkey kidney cells.

Observe: for CPE of rounded granular cells with detachment of cells from glass.

Type: by complement fixation test.

Serology
Complement fixation test.

Argentinian and Bolivian haemorrhagic fevers: are due to arenaviruses (*Junin* and *Machupo viruses* respectively). Clinically both are severe diseases with haemorrhage and renal, cardiovascular and sometimes neurological symptoms. The reservoirs of both viruses are mouse-like rodents. The Argentinian disease is rural and spreads mainly during the maize harvest; the Bolivian disease is mostly acquired in houses.

Korean haemorrhagic fever: is also known as haemorrhagic fever with renal syndrome (HFRS) — indicating the frequency with which it is accompanied by nephritis. Reported as epidemics in the Far East, it is probably the same disease as the milder nephropathia epidemica seen in Scandinavia and Eastern Europe. The cause is an orbivirus — *Hantaan virus* — of which the reservoir is small rodents.

10

Herpesvirus diseases

There are a large number of herpesviruses. Most animal species, including man, are hosts for a particular herpes virus and sometimes two or more viruses. All are morphologically identical and have the important property of remaining latent, in potentially viable form, within the cells of the host after primary infection. Latent virus persists for long periods of time — probably throughout life: some herpesviruses reactivate from time to time from the latent state to produce recurrent infection.

There are four human herpesviruses:

(1) Herpes simplex virus
(2) Varicella-zoster virus
(3) Cytomegalovirus
(4) Epstein-Barr virus.

HERPES SIMPLEX VIRUS

Herpes simplex virus is unusual among viruses in causing a wide variety of clinical syndromes: the basic lesions are vesicles but these can take many different forms.

Clinical features

Diseases due to the virus are in two categories:

(1) *Primary*: when the virus is first encountered.
(2) *Reactivation*: recurrent infections due to reactivation of latent virus.

(1) **Primary infections**

Virtually everyone becomes infected with the virus but most primary infections are symptomless. Below are listed the main clinical manifestations when primary infection is accompanied by symptoms.

(i) *Gingivo-stomatitis*: vesicles inside the mouth on the buccal mucosa and on the gums: these ulcerate and become coated with a greyish slough. Although this is the com-

monest primary disease, doubtless due to kissing as the
main mode of transmission, vesicles may be produced at
other sites, most often on the head or neck.

(ii) *Herpetic whitlow*: whitlow is due to implantation of the
virus into the fingers: the lesion produced is very similar
to a staphylococcal whitlow but the exudate is serous
rather than purulent: an occupational hazard of doctors
and nurses especially in those like anaesthetists or neuro-
surgical nurses, who deal with unconscious patients who
are intubated: infection is acquired through contamination of the hands by virus in saliva or respiratory sections.

(iii) *Conjunctivitis and keratitis*: primary herpes can involve
conjunctiva and cornea: the eyelids are usually swollen
and there are often vesicles and ulcers on them.

(iv) *Kaposi's varicelliform eruption* is a superinfection of ecze-
matous skin: mainly seen in young children, it can be a
serious disease with a significant case fatality rate.

(v) *Acute necrotising encephalitis*: herpes encephalitis is a very
rare but extremely severe disease: clinically, it presents
with the sudden onset of fever, mental confusion and
headache: the main site of infection is the temporal lobe
where the disease causes necrosis. Recently a milder form of
herpes encephalitis with a good prognosis has been described. It is uncertain if herpes encephalitis is a primary
infection or a reactivation.

(vi) *Genital herpes*: a vesicular eruption of the genital area due
to a variant of the virus known as herpes simplex virus
type 2: type 2 virus is antigenically and biologically
slightly different (although also similar in many properties) to the more common type 1 herpes simplex virus
which infects the head and neck; genital herpes is usually
sexually transmitted.

(vii) *Neonatal infection*: severe generalised infection in neonates is usually acquired from a primary genital infection
in the mother when no maternal antibody is present for
the protection of the child: affected infants have jaundice,
hepatosplenomegaly, thrombocytopaenia and large vesicular lesions on the skin: there is a high case fatality rate:
usually due to herpes simplex virus type 2.

(viii) *Generalised infection* is a very rare manifestation of primary infection in adults with type 1 virus: *herpes hepatitis*
has also been described.

LATENCY

After, or possibly during primary infection, the virus travels from the site of infection in the mouth to the trigeminal ganglia. The mode of travel is unknown but is probably via the nerves. Virus remains in the ganglia in a potentially viable state and in a proportion of people, reactivates to cause recurrent infection. Even in the absence of recurrent infection virus can be isolated from the trigeminal ganglia in most normal people. The state of the virus in the ganglion cells is unknown but it is almost certainly not present as intact virions: the most popular current theory is that latent virus is probably in the form of virus DNA integrated into the cellular chromosomes. In genital herpes, type 2 virus becomes latent in the sacral ganglia.

Reactivation of virus is provoked by various stimuli including common colds, sunlight (possibly a result of exposure to ultra-violet light), pneumonia, stress, menstruation, etc. Reactivation recurs sporadically, sometimes often, throughout life.

Neutralising antibody is formed after primary infection but — surprisingly — does not prevent reactivation: this may be because herpes is protected from serum antibody as it travels within the axons of sensory nerves to the sites of recurrent infection. Reactivation does not stimulate a rise in titre of herpes antibody.

(2) **Clinical manifestations of reactivation:**
   (i) *Cold sores*: or vesicles round mucocutaneous junctions of nose and mouth are the most common: the vesicles progress to pustules with crust formation: the virus appears to travel down the maxillary or mandibular branches of the trigeminal nerve to reach areas of the skin supplied by these nerves; recurrent herpetic vesicles are seen — but more rarely — at other sites on the skin: genital lesions may also recur and these are due to type 2 virus.
   (ii) *Keratitis*: reactivation less commonly affects the eye: recurrent lesions are usually restricted to the cornea and the conjunctiva is not involved: virus probably reaches the cornea via the ophthalmic branch of the trigeminal nerve: lesions take the form of a branching or *dendritic ulcer*: if recurrence is frequent, scarring developes and in a few cases the disease progresses to a severe, destructive uveitis.
   (iii) *Immunosuppressive therapy*: especially in renal transplant patients is sometimes associated with severe, extensive cold

sores; usually in the mouth, these may be necrotic and spread to involve large areas of the face and into the oesophagus.

Epidemiology

Infectivity: Herpes simplex is not a very infectious virus and there are, for example, no outbreaks of herpes infections in the community.

Spread: by close personal contact, e.g. kissing (type 1 virus), sexual intercourse (type 2 virus).

Sources: generally people with herpetic lesions; however, carriers of the latent virus from time to time secrete virus in their saliva without any symptoms and this may act as a source of (undetected) infection.

Age: infection is most common in childhood and is usually symptomless: there is another peak in incidence during adolescence due to kissing as contact with the opposite sex increases.

Infection: is virtually universal in human populations and in elderly people the incidence of antibody (indicating previous infection) is almost 100 per cent.

Virology
1. Roughly spherical particle with cubic symmetry, medium size — 100 nm, with 162 projecting hollow-cored capsomeres; many of the particles are surrounded by a loose envelope of material partially derived from the host cell (Fig. 10.1).
2. Double-stranded DNA.
3. Two types of virus — 1 and 2: types 1 and 2 share antigens in common (group-specific) but possess type-specific antigens also: although their DNA shows some homology, the two types of DNA can be readily distinguished by restriction enzyme analysis. Virus-specified proteins of the two viruses are produced in approximately equal numbers but can be distinguished by differences in their molecular weights when separated by electrophoresis in polyacrylamide gels.
4. Grows in various tissue cultures with characteristic CPE with ballooning and rounding of cells.
5. Grows on chorio-allantoic membrane with production of tiny white pocks.
6. Pathogenic for laboratory animals causing encephalitis.

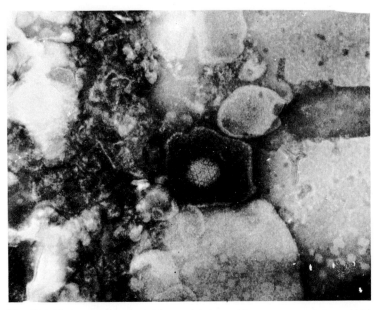

Fig. 10.1 Herpes simplex virus. The particle has cubic symmetry and the capsid is composed of hollow-cored capsomeres. There is a loose, baggy envelope. × 108 000. (Photograph by Dr E.A.C. Follett.)

Diagnosis

Isolation

Specimens: vesicle fluid, skin swab, saliva, conjunctival fluid, corneal scrapings, brain biopsy.

Inoculate: tissue cultures, e.g. BHK21 (a hamster kidney cell line), human embryo lung cells.

Observe: for CPE of rounded cells.

Type: by neutralisation test with standard antiserum.

Serology
Complement fixation test, useful for diagnosing primary infections; difficult to interpret in recurrent infections because of high levels of existing antibody and because recurrences usually do not cause a rise in titre.

Chemotherapy (see also Chapter 14)

Idoxuridine (0.1% solution) is regularly used topically in the treatment of herpes keratitis. Herpetic skin lesions and whitlows can be treated topically with stronger solutions (i.e. 5% — or 40% for whitlows — in dimethyl sulphoxide).

Vidarabine: has been used intravenously in severe herpes. However, early trials suggest that *acyclovir* will be the most effective anti-herpes drug both topically and systemically.

VARICELLA-ZOSTER VIRUS

Varicella (chickenpox) and zoster (shingles — but also sometimes called 'herpes zoster') are different diseases due to the same virus. *Varicella is the primary illness.*
Zoster is a recurrent manifestation of infection.

VARICELLA

Clinical features

Varicella is a common childhood fever. There is a mild febrile illness with a characteristic vesicular rash; the vesicles appear in successive waves so that lesions of different age are present together; the vesicles (in which there are giant cells) develop into pustules.

The varicella rash has a close resemblance to that seen in smallpox which has been modified by vaccination.

Complications are rare: post-infectious encephalomyelitis, haemorrhagic (fulminating) varicella; in adults pneumonia is a relatively common and serious complication and may be followed by permanent pulmonary calcification.

Congenital varicella is exceedingly rare: maternal varicella in early pregnancy is occasionally followed by a syndrome in the infant of limb hypoplasia, muscular atrophy and cerebral and psychomotor retardation.

Perinatal or neonatal varicella: maternal varicella near the time of delivery may affect the child: if the mother contracts varicella more than 5 days before delivery, the disease in the child is usually mild: this is because the child's disease is modified by placentally-transmitted early maternal antibody: when maternal varicella is within 5 days of delivery, there is not time for maternal antibody to be produced and to cross the placenta, and the child is liable to develop severe disease.

Immunity: attack is followed by solid and long lasting immunity to varicella — but *not* to zoster.

Epidemiology

Seasonal distribution: highest incidence is in autumn and winter.

Spread: via nose and mouth by droplet infection from infectious saliva; virus is also present in skin lesions.

Varicella is an epidemic contagious disease; it may be acquired by contact with cases either of varicella or less commonly of zoster.

Zoster

The disease is *due to reactivation of virus* latent in dorsal root or cranial nerve ganglia following — and usually many years after — childhood varicella.

Mainly affects adults: clinically there is an eruption of *crops of painful vesicles* in areas of skin corresponding in distribution to one or more sensory nerves; the most commonly affected are the thoracic nerves and less commonly the cranial — notably the ophthalmic — nerves.

When dorsal root ganglia are involved there is a segmental rash which extends from the middle of the back in a horizontal strip round the side of the chest wall — 'a belt of roses from hell'.

When the ophthalmic nerve of the trigeminal ganglion is affected the rash is distributed within the skin supplied by that nerve depending on the roots affected. This may cause a sharply demarcated area of lesions down one side of the forehead and scalp: in about half the patients, there are lesions in the eye.

Ramsay Hunt syndrome is a rare form of zoster: the eruption is on the tympanic membrane and the external auditory canal and there is often a facial nerve palsy.

Residual neuralgia — which may be severe — often follows zoster in the elderly.

Neurological signs are sometimes seen, e.g. paralysis.

Note: Virus is present in both the skin lesions and in the corresponding dorsal root ganglion

Epidemiology
Zoster — unlike varicella — is not acquired by contact with cases of either varicella or zoster — although it may give rise to cases of varicella in susceptible contacts.
Cases are *sporadic* and there is *no seasonal distribution.*

Virology
1. One serological type; in the electron microscope the particle is that of a typical herpes virus and is morphologically identical to that of herpes simplex.
2. Grows slowly in tissue cultures of human cells (e.g. human embryo lung or thyroid tissue cultures) with CPE but *the virus remains cell associated*, i.e. no free virus is released into the medium. This has greatly hampered investigation of the virus.

Diagnosis

Serology
Complement fixation test: unlike reactivations of herpes simplex, zoster usually causes a rise in antibody titre.

Isolation
Rarely attempted.

CYTOMEGALOVIRUS

Cytomegalovirus diseases are examples of *'opportunistic infections'*, i.e. the virus rarely causes disease unless precipitating factors are present which lower the normal resistance of the host.

Symptomless infections are common: about 50% of the adult population has antibody to the virus almost always without developing any symptoms of disease.

Latency: the virus is known to reactivate from the latent state in, for example, renal transplant patients on immunosuppressive therapy: the site of latency is uncertain but is probably polymorphonuclear leucocytes or lymphocytes.
There are two types of disease due to cytomegalovirus:

1. Congenital infection

Neonates may be born infected with cytomegalovirus acquired *in utero* from mothers with symptomless infections in whom virus is excreted in urine or saliva. There is a spectrum of disease in the infants from inapparent infection, to a mild disease (although this may be followed by mental retardation) to a severe generalised disease known as cytomegalic inclusion disease (CID).

Severe, generalised infection (CID)

Signs and symptoms: affected infants have jaundice, hepatosplenomegaly, blood dyscrasias such as thrombocytopenia and haemolytic anaemia; the brain is usually involved causing microcephaly and motor disorders; surviving infants are usually mentally retarded. Cytomegalovirus is probably the cause of about 10% of cases of microcephaly.

Affected organs: show characteristic enlarged cells (hence the prefix 'cytomegalo') with large intranuclear or 'owl's eye' inclusions; these are found mainly in the salivary glands, liver, lungs and kidneys.

Severe generalized disease is relatively rare: most congenital infections are less immediately serious but may also be followed by *mental retardation*.

2. Postnatal infection

Hepatitis

In children, cytomegalovirus causes *hepatitis* with enlargement of the liver and disturbance of liver function tests; jaundice may or may not be present.

Infectious mononucleosis

In adults, infection may take the form of an illness like infectious mononucleosis but with a negative Paul Bunnell reaction and no lymphadenopathy or pharyngitis. There is fever, hepatitis and lymphocytosis with atypical lymphocytes in the peripheral blood; the syndrome is sometimes seen after transfusion with fresh unfrozen blood — presumably cytomegalovirus, which may occasionally be present in the donor's blood, is normally inactivated by storage at 4°C.

Infection in the immunocompromised

Disseminated infection is also seen when *immunosuppressive therapy* or *severe debilitating disease*, such as neoplasm, is present to lower the host's resistance. There are usually widespread lesions involving lungs as well as other organs and tissues, e.g. adrenals, liver and alimentary tract. This is an occasional complication of renal transplantation;

Renal transplant patients are subject to frequent infections with cytomegalovirus — probably mainly reactivations of latent virus — but these are not always associated with signs or symptoms of disease. *Pneumonitis* and, rarely, *retinitis* due to cytomegalovirus have been reported in transplant patients.

Virology
1. Electron microscopy — a typical herpes virus particle.
2. Grows slowly in cultures of human embryo lung cells with characteristic CPE and intranuclear 'owl's eye' inclusions.

Diagnosis

Isolation

Specimens: urine, throat swab.

Inoculate: human embryo lung cell cultures.

Observe: for characteristic CPE of swollen cells; this may take from 2 to 3 weeks to appear.

Serology
Complement fixation test, immunofluorescence.

Demonstration
Of typical intranuclear 'owl's eye' inclusion in cells of urinary sediment or other tissues.

EPSTEIN-BARR (EB) VIRUS

Epstein-Barr virus is named after the two virologists who first observed it when examining cultures of lymphoblasts from Burkitt's lymphoma in the electron microscope.

EB virus infection is widespread in human populations and most people have antibody to it by the time they reach adulthood.

Most infections are symptomless: especially if acquired during childhood; if infection is delayed until adult life there is greater likelihood of disease; this takes the form of *infectious mononucleosis* or glandular fever.

Persistence of virus: EB virus persists in latent form within lymphocytes following primary infection: the virus is present in lymphocytes in the form of viral DNA — both free in the cytoplasm and integrated into the cellular chromosone.

Burkitt's lymphoma: the virus may cause this cancer of the lymphoid tissues which is common in African children (see Chapter 16).

INFECTIOUS MONONUCLEOSIS (glandular fever)

Clinical features

Incubation period: is long — from 4 to 7 weeks.

Route of infection: close or intimate contact, e.g. kissing; the virus has been demonstrated in cells in salivary secretions. The disease is most prevalent amongst young adults, especially student populations.

Signs and symptoms: low-grade fever with generalized lymphadenopathy and sore throat due to exudative tonsillitis; malaise, anorexia and tiredness to a severe degree are characteristic features; splenomegaly is common and most cases have abnormal liver function tests; a proportion have palpable enlargement of the liver and frank jaundice is not uncommon.

Mononucleosis: or — more correctly — a relative and absolute lymphocytosis is a diagnostic feature; at least 10% and usually more of the lymphocytes are atypical with enlarged misshapen nuclei and more cytoplasm than normal; the atypical lymphocytes are both B and T cells.

Paul Bunnell test: infectious mononucleosis is characteristically associated with the appearance in the blood of heterophil antibody to sheep erythrocytes; this antibody can be removed by absorption with ox erythrocytes but not by absorption with guinea pig kidney. This differential absorption and the haemagglutination test with sheep erythrocytes constitutes the Paul Bunnell test and is diagnostic of infectious mononucleosis: development of other non-specific antibodies (e.g. rheumatoid factor and anti-i cold agglutinin) are a feature of the disease.

EB virus antibody: is also produced during infection although antibody may be present before symptoms develop; the presence of EB virus-specific IgM is a useful confirmatory diagnostic test.

Duration: in most cases of infectious mononucleosis symptoms last from 2 to 3 weeks but, in a proportion, the illness may persist for weeks or even months.

Virology
1. Electron microscopy — a typical herpesvirus
2. Grows only in suspension cultures of human lymphoblasts and usually only a proportion of cells carry or replicate the virus.
3. Virus can be detected by electron microscopy or immunofluorescence.
4. EB virus can be detected or isolated by its ability to 'transform' normal human lymphocytes into a continuously dividing line of cells.

Diagnosis

Serology
1. Paul Bunnell test.
2. Demonstration of EB virus-specific IgM or rising titre (IgG) to EB virus by immunofluorescence; the antibody tested is that directed against the viral capsid antigen.

Haematology
Demonstration of atypical lymphocytes in the peripheral blood.

11

Mumps, measles, rubella

Mumps, measles and rubella are, with varicella, the common childhood fevers. Measles has been, at least partially controlled by vaccination and this has altered its traditional epidemiology. Rubella vaccination is aimed at protecting against the risk of fetal infection while not interfering with naturally-acquired immunity. An effective mumps vaccine is available but is not in general use.

MUMPS

Clinical features

Incubation period: relatively long — 18 to 21 days.

Clinically: a febrile illness with inflammation of salivary glands causing characteristitic swelling of parotid and submaxillary glands.

Neurological complications are also not uncommon; these usually take the form of aseptic meningitis or meningoencephalitis; occasionally there is muscular weakness or paralysis. Neurological syndromes due to mumps virus are not accompanied by parotitis in 50% of cases. *Nerve deafness* is a rare complication.

Other complications: orchitis, pancreatitis and — very rarely — *oophoritis* and *thyroiditis* are seen in association with mumps; about 20% of adult males who contract mumps develop orchitis.

Immunity: an attack is followed by solid and long-lasting immunity; second attacks are very rare.

Mumps is a generalised infection by a virus with a predilection for the CNS (neurotropism) and for glandular tissue.

Epidemiology

Spread is by droplet infection with infectious saliva via the nose and mouth.

Seasonal distribution: the highest incidence is in the spring.

Age distribution: commonest in children aged from 5 to 15 years but is not uncommon in young adults and outbreaks have been reported in recruit populations.

Infectiousness: lower than measles; as a result infection in childhood is not as common as with measles and a significant proportion of adults are non-immune.

Importance is mainly due to the relative frequency of neurological complications especially when mumps infects adults; mumps is an important cause of aseptic meningitis.

Epidemics of mumps last about 2 years and are followed by a year when the incidence of infection is low; another period of high incidence then appears.

Virology

1. Paramyxovirus, one serological type.
2. RNA virus.
3. Enveloped particles, rather large in size — 110 to 170 nm; helical symmetry.
4. Haemagglutinates fowl erythrocytes.
5. Grows in amniotic cavity of chick embryo and in monkey kidney and other tissue cultures with haemadsorption.

Diagnosis

Serology (widely used)
Complement fixation test: Two antigens are used:
1. 'S' or soluble antigen (the nucleoprotein core of the virus particle);
2. 'V' or viral antigen (found on the surface of the virus particle).

Antibody to 'S' antigen tends to diminish sooner than antibody to 'V' antigen; it can therefore be a useful indicator of recent infection.

'V' antibody usually persists for years.

Isolation (not so useful as serology)

Specimens: saliva — or CSF in neurological disease.

Inoculate: monkey kidney tissue cultures or amniotic cavity of chick embryo.

Observe: tissue cultures for haemadsorption of fowl erythrocytes; *chick embryo* for appearance of haemagglutinin for fowl erythrocytes in amniotic fluid.

Type virus: by inhibition of haemadsorption or haemagglutination with standard antiserum.

Vaccine
A mumps vaccine has recently become available.

Contains: live attenuated virus grown in chick embryo cells.

Administered: in one dose subcutaneously.

Protection: apparently good.

Reactions: occasionally mild fever.

MEASLES

Clinical features
Measles is the most common of the childhood fevers; in uncomplicated cases it is a mild disease but complications are relatively frequent.
   Measles starts with prodromal respiratory symptoms such as nasal discharge and suffusion of the eyes.

The characteristic illness of measles follows; the main features are fever — which may be high — with a maculopapular rash lasting from two to five days.

Immunity following measles is life-long.

Complications

Respiratory infections: are the most common and are seen in about 4% of patients; these include bronchitis, bronchiolitis, croup and bronchopneumonia; *otitis media* is also seen in about 2.5% of cases. Before the advent of the antibiotics these infections were more frequent and were largely responsible for the mortality associated with measles.

Rarer complications are encephalitis and giant cell pneumonia.
Two types of encephalitis are seen:
1. *Encephalitis or post-infectious encephalomyelitis*: a serious condition which follows measles in about one in every 1000 cases; the mortality rate is about 50% and many of the survivors have residual neurological symptoms. Encephalitis commonly presents with drowsiness, vomiting, headache and convulsions.
2. *Subacute sclerosing panencephalitis*: A very rare but severe, chronic, neurological disease seen in children and young adults. The presenting symptoms are of personality and behavioural changes with intellectual impairment; the disease progresses to convulsions, myoclonic movements and increasing neurological deterioration leading to coma and death. Due to persistent infection with measles virus following primary and usually uncomplicated measles several years previously; affected children have high titres of measles antibody in their serum and both IgM and IgG measles-specific antibody in the CSF.

At post mortem, there are numerous intranuclear inclusions throughout the brain: measles virus has been grown from brain tissue.

Giant cell pneumonia: a rare complication, seen mainly in children with chronic debilitating diseases; it is due to direct invasion of the lungs by measles virus and is usually fatal: there are numerous multinucleated giant cells in the lungs at post-mortem.

Epidemiology

The attack rate in measles is high: virtually everybody in Britain under the age of 15 years has had the disease or — nowadays — been vaccinated against it. When the disease has been introduced into isolated communities where measles is not endemic and the entire population is susceptible, attack rates of more than 99% have been recorded.

Spread is by inhalation of respiratory secretions from patients in the early stages of the disease.

Epidemics: measles in Britain used to appear in epidemics every second year; this is probably because in two years sufficient new susceptible hosts had been born into the community for the virus to become epidemic again; in non-epidemic years, measles was endemic but the number of cases was lower than in epidemic years.

The introduction of measles vaccine has caused a marked reduction in the incidence both of measles and measles encephalitis.

In countries like Britain, where there is little poverty and malnutrition, measles is a mild disease with a low mortality rate.

In under-developed countries, e.g. West Africa, measles is a severe disease and a serious cause of death in childhood.

Virology
1. Paramyxovirus, one serological type.
2. RNA virus.
3. Enveloped particles, rather large size, 120 to 250 nm; helical symmetry.
4. Haemagglutinates and haemolyses monkey erythrocytes.
5. Grows in human amnion cells with syncytial CPE of multinucleated giant cells.

Diagnosis
Confirmation can be obtained by isolating the virus in human amnion tissue cultures or serologically by complement fixation test, but the disease has a characteristic clinical picture and this is rarely necessary.

Vaccine
Measles vaccination has been introduced to reduce the morbidity due to respiratory complications and the risk of encephalitis. Routine immunisation in the second year of life is now officially recommended in Britain.

Contains: virus attenuated by passage in tissue cultures of chick embryo fibroblasts.

Administered: in one dose subcutaneously.

Protection: good: however, although the immunity conferred is apparently long-lasting, some cases of atypical measles have been reported in adolescents who had been vaccinated as children: this suggests that the immunity may not be so long-lasting as that following natural infection. It would be potentially serious if vaccination in childhood left some people unprotected in adult life when the natural disease is often more severe.

Reactions: reactions such as fever and rash are fairly common but are milder than in natural measles.

Safety: vaccinated children are not infectious to others although virus multiplies in their bodies.

Normal immunoglobulin

Normal immunoglobulin is derived from pooled human sera and therefore contains measles antibody: it has been used to confer passive immunity to infants and other unusually susceptible individuals who have been in contact with cases of measles.

RUBELLA

Rubella is a mild childhood fever but if infection is contracted in early pregnancy the virus can cause congenital abnormalities in the fetus.

Clinical features

Rubella is a mild febrile illness with a macular rash which spreads down from the face and behind the ears; there is usually pharyngitis and enlargement of the cervical — and especially the posterior cervical — lymph glands.

Virus is commonly present in both blood and pharyngeal secretions; virus is excreted during the incubation period for up to seven days before the appearance of the rash.

Many infections are symptomless.

Complications are rare. These include post-infectious encephalomyelitis, thrombocytopenic purpura and arthralgia or painful joints.

Epidemiology

Rubella mainly attacks children under 15 years of age but many children reach adult life without being infected and infection in adults is not uncommon; about 15% of women of child-bearing age have not been infected and are therefore non-immune.

Infection is endemic in the community with epidemics every few years: the most extensive outbreak recorded was in the USA in 1964 when there were 1 800 000 cases.

The teratogenic properties of the virus were first discovered in Australia in 1941: it was noticed that an increase in the number of cases of congenital cataract had followed an epidemic of rubella:

affected infants had been born to mothers with a history of rubella in early pregnancy and it was concluded that early maternal rubella can cause congenital defects in the offspring.

Congenital defects follow rubella only in the first 16 weeks of pregnancy; after that rubella does not damage the fetus.

The main defects are a triad of:

Cataract

Nerve deafness

Cardiac abnormalities (e.g. patent ductus arteriosus, ventricular septal defect, pulmonary artery stenosis, Fallot's tetralogy.)

The affected infants have various disorders due to generalised infection which, together with the defects, are known as *the rubella syndrome*; these are:

Hepatosplenomegaly

Thrombocytopenic purpura

Low birth weight

Mental retardation

Jaundice

Anaemia

Lesions in the metaphyses of the long bones.

The type and frequency of defect vary with the time of infection. Multiple severe defects are seen after rubella in the first six weeks of pregnancy.

The incidence of major defect after maternal rubella in the first three months of pregnancy has been found to be 16%; the comparable figure in a control group was 2.3%. Maternal rubella was also associated with a higher proportion of abortions and stillbirths.

The total incidence of deafness increased to 19% when children exposed to rubella *in utero* were examined at the age of 3 to 5 years. The incidence of both deafness and defective vision further increased as the children grew up — probably due to easier recognition of these defects in older children.

Subacute sclerosing parencephalitis has been reported as a rare, late complication of congenital rubella.

Infants with the rubella syndrome have IgM antibody to rubella virus and therefore are immunologically competent (the maternal antibody which crosses the placenta is IgG antibody).

Antibody protects against re-infection and second attacks appear to be rare (some reported second attacks may have been due to other infections misdiagnosed as rubella since rubella is not a particularly distinctive illness).

Virology
1. Classified as a non-arthropod-borne togavirus, one serological type.
2. RNA virus.
3. Pleomorphic-enveloped particles, medium size — 50 to 75 nm; helical symmetry.
4. Haemagglutinates bird erythrocytes, e.g. from day-old chicks.
5. Grows in a rabbit kidney cell line — RK 13 with production of CPE and in other tissue cultures but without CPE.

Diagnosis
Laboratory diagnosis is now widely used for confirmation of the diagnosis of rubella — usually in a pregnant woman or in suspected congenital rubella; also used to detect non-immune women who may be offered vaccination.

Serology

Haemagglutination-inhibition test: the most sensitive technique for detecting rubella antibody: active rubella (e.g. in pregnancy) is best diagnosed by demonstration of a rising titre of IgG. Specimens need only be 3 days apart.

IgM antibody: recent infection with rubella virus can also be diagnosed by the demonstration of IgM rubella antibody in a single sample of blood; this is because IgM antibody is only present for a short time after acute infection. IgM antibody is detected by fractionating serum on a sucrose gradient to separate IgM from IgG antibody; the fraction containing IgM antibodies is then tested by haemagglutination-inhibition for rubella-specific antibody. This technique is especially useful in pregnant women when only stationary titres of rubella antibody can be detected by standard tests; it can also be used to diagnose congenital rubella in infants.

Complement fixation test: but titres of antibody are lower and do not persist so long as haemagglutination-inhibiting antibody.

Radial immune haemolysis: widely used for detecting immunity in pregnant women or in women at special risk e.g. children's nurses, schoolteachers: it does not measure antibody titre and is not suitable for the diagnosis of rubella.

Vaccination

Live attenuated virus vaccine

Contains: virus attenuated by passage in tissue culture; virus is grown in either primary rabbit kidney cells or WI38 human embryo fibroblasts.

Administered: one dose subcutaneously.

Protection: good, immunity so far appears to be long-lasting.

Reactions: mild; sometimes slight fever and rash; mild arthralgia is seen occasionally in adult females.

Viral excretion: Many vaccinees excrete virus from the nasopharynx but are apparently non-infectious to contacts.

Indications: schoolgirls aged 11 to 13 years; non-immune women of childbearing age (who must avoid pregnancy for three months after vaccination).

Contra-indication: Pregnant women should not be given vaccine since the vaccine virus is capable of crossing the placenta to infect the fetus.

Note: rubella vaccination has been in force in Britain for nine years; it is still not certain if it is succeeding in reducing the incidence of congenital rubella; perhaps as the first schoolgirls who were vaccinated grow up and marry a protective effect may become more apparent.

Passive immunisation with rubella-specific immunoglobulin may have some slight attenuating or prophylactic effect in rubella. It may be considered for use in maternal rubella if termination is refused.

12

Poxvirus diseases

Smallpox was one of the most severe viral diseases with a considerable mortality rate. Jenner showed in the eighteenth century that smallpox could be prevented by vaccination. A discovery which meant that since man is the only host for the virus, complete eradication of the disease was theoretically possible. Happily, this has now been accomplished by the World Health Organisation.

Clinical features
Smallpox is a systemic viral infection with a characteristic severe vesicular rash; the rash affects the face and extremities more than the trunk (centrifugal distribution).

Incubation period: 12 days.

First symptoms: fever and malaise for about four days.

Rash appears on the 16th day from contact; the earliest lesions are maculo-papules which become vesicles and then progress to pustules.
 There are two clinically distinct forms of smallpox:
1. *Variola major* (or classical smallpox) the most severe form of the disease.
 The mortality rate is high–32% in unvaccinated subjects.
2. *Alastrim* (or variola minor) A milder form of the disease: mortality rate–0.25%

Epidemiology

Patients are infectious from the 11th day or 12th day after contact with maximum infectivity during the first week of illness.

Source of infection: mainly virus shed from the respiratory tract.

Route of infection: by inhalation

Virology
The pox group of viruses includes the human viruses variola (and the related alastrim) and molluscum contagiosum: there are numerous animal poxviruses such as cowpox which was used by Jenner for vaccination against smallpox: the origin of vaccinia — the virus now used for vaccination — is unclear.

The following properties are common to poxviruses:
1. DNA viruses.
2. Large brick-shaped particles 200 to 300 nm (Fig. 12.1)
3. Most produce pocks on chorio-allantoic membrane of chick embryo.
4. Grow in monkey kidney and other tissue cultures (with CPE with characteristic 'ballooning' of the cells).
5. Haemagglutinate fowl erythrocytes.

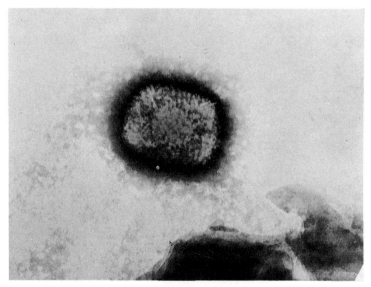

Fig. 12.1 Vaccinia virus. Brick-shaped particles with complex symmetry. × 90 000. (Photograph by Dr E.A.C. Follett.)

Diagnosis of smallpox

Specimens: scrapings from maculo-papules, vesicle fluid, crusts.
1. *Direct demonstration of virus*: Electron microscopy: smears are examined for characteristic poxvirus particles.

2. *Dectection of pox group viral antigen in skin lesions*: serological tests detect only common pox group antigens:
   (i) *Complement fixation test*:
   (ii) *Gel diffusion tests*:
3. *Isolation of virus* The only method of distinguishing between variola and vaccinia viruses.

   Inoculate: chorio-allantoic membrane of chick embryo.

   Observe. 2 to 3 days for characteristic pocks:

   variola major: small white pocks (Fig. 12.2): able to grow at 38.3°C as well as at the usual temperature of incubation of 35–36°C.

   alastrim: small white pocks, do not grow at 38.3°C.

   vaccinia: large grey fluffy pocks with necrotic centres.

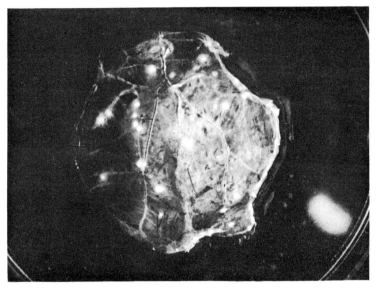

Fig. 12.2 Chorio-allantoic membrane of chick embryo showing small white pearl-like pocks formed by variola (smallpox) virus. (Photograph by Prof. C.R. Madeley.)

Vaccination

In 1798 Edward Jenner reported that artificial inoculation of cowpox protected against smallpox. Cowpox is a natural infection of cows which is sometimes transmitted to the hands of milkers from infected udders.

Vaccinia virus now used as smallpox vaccine differs considerably from cowpox virus: it may be a hybrid, derived from cowpox by recombination with other poxviruses or may even be a different virus (e.g. horsepox).

There is a close immunological relationship between vaccinia and variola viruses so that infection with vaccinia provides immunity against variola. Smallpox vaccine is prepared from the vesicles which result from the inoculation of the abdominal wall of sheep or calves with vaccinia virus.

Inoculation is carried out by making multiple light pressures with a Hagedorn needle through a drop of vaccine placed on the skin of the upper arm.

Primary or revaccination vaccinia: a vesicle appears at the 7th to 8th day and the reaction reaches maximal intensity at the 12th day.

Accelerated reactions: true reactions and common in partially immune people; the vesicle appears at the 4th or 5th day with maximal intensity about the 7th day.

Immediate reactions: are due to allergy to some constituent of the vaccine; sometimes an early vesicle forms but usually there is only a papule seen at the 2nd or 3rd day with some surrounding erythema. Immediate or negative reactions are not evidence of pre-existing immunity.

Protection conferred: solid immunity against smallpox lasts for about three years after vaccination: immunity wanes at a variable rate over the next 7 to 10 years.

Complications

There are two main kinds of complications after vaccination:

1. *Encephalitis*: or post-infectious encephalomyelitis. Incidence — one per 100 000 vaccinations.
2. *Generalised vaccinia*: seen mainly in infants and clinically divided into three types:

    (i) *Mild generalised vaccinia*: the most common complication in which the vaccine virus causes lesions outwith the vaccinated area; low mortality rate; incidence is about one per 25 000 vaccinations. Sometimes *the lesions are numerous and severe* — especially in immuno-compromised patients; in these cases the mortality rate is high.

    (ii) *Eczema vaccinatum*: or Kaposi's varicelliform eruption (which may also be due to herpes simplex virus) superinfection of eczema; usually transmitted from vaccinated siblings.

(iii) *Chronic progressive vaccinia* or *vaccinia gangrenosa*: a very rare and serious complication in which the vaccination gradually extends locally with severe and progressive tissue necrosis. Some — but not all — cases have a defect in cell-mediated immunity.

Pregnant women: should not be vaccinated because of the danger of severe fetal infection or *prenatal vaccinia*.

Eradication
In 1967 the World Health Organisation embarked on a Smallpox Eradication campaign. This was based on a policy of 'search and containment' i.e. isolation of cases and the tracing and vaccination of contacts. There was continuing and long-term surveillance of previously endemic areas before these were declared smallpox-free. The main endemic areas were India, Pakistan and Bangladesh and, in Africa, Ethiopia and Somalia. Smallpox has now been eradicated from them and the World Health Organisation declared the world free from smallpox in May 1980.

OTHER POXVIRUS DISEASES

Molluscum contagiosum
A low grade infection in man characterised by reddish, waxy papules on the skin — most often seen in the axilla or on the trunk. It is a fairly common infection in children and is spread by close contact, e.g. at swimming baths; the lesions contain numerous poxvirus particles which can be seen in the electron microscope; the lesions resolve spontaneously in 4 to 6 weeks.

Orf or contagious pustular dermatitis
An infection of sheep and goats: occasionally transmitted to hands of animal workers causing chronic granulomatous lesions; diagnosed by characteristic oval particles in electron microscope with criss-cross surface banding.

Paravaccinia or pseudocowpox
The virus appears to be identical with orf virus: it causes lesions on udders of cows and is occasionally transmitted to hands of animal workers.

Monkeypox
This is a disease resembling mild smallpox which is due to a natural

pox virus of monkeys; it is seen in Africa among people with frequent contact with monkeys.

Tanapox
This virus is probably also acquired from contact with monkeys
and, in humans, produces scanty vesicular lesions on the skin
which do not progress to pustules. Epidemics have been reported in
East Africa.

13

Viral hepatitis

Hepatitis is a complication of infection with several different viruses, e.g. cytomegalovirus, EB virus, and yellow fever virus. However, the most common forms of viral hepatitis are hepatitis A, hepatitis B and the recently discovered non-A, non-B hepatitis. Hepatitis A is a childhood enteric infection but hepatitis B is mainly transmitted parenterally e.g. by blood transfusion. Non-A, non-B hepatitis includes several forms of the disease and is spread both parenterally and by the faecal-oral route.

Below are the clinical features of these three diseases:

Clinical features

Hepatitis A, hepatitis B and non-A, non-B hepatitis: have similar signs and symptoms and can usually be differentiated only by tests or history of exposure. The most striking symptom is *jaundice* with dark bile-containing urine and pale stools — classical features of obstructive jaundice; liver function tests are abnormal with raised levels of serum aspartate amino transaminase (AST) and serum alanine amino transaminase (ALT); there is usually a low grade fever with nausea — which may be severe — and vomiting. Patients commonly feel tired and depressed for weeks or even months after the acute attack.

Anicteric hepatitis: is a common form of viral hepatitis in which, although liver function tests are abnormal, damage to the liver is insufficient to cause frank jaundice.

Symptomless infection: is common.

Arthralgia and rash: are seen in the prodromal stage of hepatitis B; these are thought to be serum-sickness-like symptoms due to immune complexes formed between hepatitis virus and specific antibody.

Fulminant hepatic failure is a rare but serious complication of hepatitis. In this, centrilobular confluent necrosis leads to massive hepatic necrosis; the patients develop progressive liver failure and the mortality rate is high. A particular problem in pregnancy with non-A, non-B hepatitis.

Viraemia: virus is present in the blood during the acute phase; persistent viraemia is common in hepatitis B but not in hepatitis A in which virus is usually cleared rapidly from the blood after the acute illness.

Virus in faeces: the stools are infectious in hepatitis A; virus is not present in faeces in hepatitis B.
Hepatitis A and B have been extensively studied: the main differences between them are listed in Table 13.1.

Table 13.1 Main differences between hepatitis A and hepatitis B

	Hepatitis A	Hepatitis B
Incubation period	2 to 6 weeks	2 to 5 months
Transmission	faecal-oral	parenteral: close personal contact
Age	mainly schoolchildren	mainly young adult males
Seasonal incidence	autumn and winter	none
Onset	acute	insidious
Clinically	milder	generally more severe
Hepatitis B antigen in blood	no	yes
Persistent infection	no	yes
Mortality rate	0.1–0.2%	low but higher than in hepatitis A

HEPATITIS A

Epidemiology

World-wide in distribution: endemic in most countries, more common in rural than urban communities. Epidemics appear from time to time, some of which are associated with sewage contamination of food or water.

Age incidence: mainly affects children aged 5 to 15 years but epidemics are seen in military recruit populations and children's institutions; food-borne outbreaks may involve adults predominantly.

Alimentary infection: the site of entry and of primary multiplication of the virus is the alimentary tract; virus is excreted in the faeces for about 2 weeks before the onset of jaundice but for only a few days after the development of symptoms. Hepatitis is a complication due to spread of virus to the liver (where it replicates in the hepatocytes) in what is primarily an enteric infection. Antibody to hepatitis A virus appears at the time of onset of jaundice — initially IgM with later but longer persisting IgG.

There are two main routes of infection:

1. *Case-to-case spread* via the faecal-oral route, the most common route of spread of the disease; symptomless excretors may be an important — because undetected — source of infection.

2. *Via contaminated food and water*: numerous outbreaks have been described due to contamination of food-stuffs by a food-handler who is excreting virus or to pollution of water by infected sewage. The largest outbreak was in Delhi in 1955–56 where there were 29 000 cases following contamination of the main city water supply by sewage. *Raw oysters and shellfish* which have become contaminated by growing in sewage-polluted water have been responsible for several large outbreaks.

Decline: there has been a striking decline in the incidence of hepatitis A in Europe (and especially in Britain) over the past 10 years. This seems to be due to some block in the normal faecal-oral route of transmission in children. The decrease in incidence has not been observed in underdeveloped or tropical countries.

Virology
1. RNA (single-stranded) virus.
2. Small spherical particles, 27–30 nm.
3. Relatively heat-resistant i.e. withstands 60°C for 30 minutes.
4. Does not grow in tissue culture by ordinary methods: some limited multiplication of laboratory adapted strains has been demonstrated in primate cells: there is no CPE.
5. Pathogenic for chimpanzees and other primates e.g. marmosets.

Diagnosis
1. *Serology* Radio-immune Assay: detection of virus-specific IgM.
2. *Demonstration of virus* in stools by electron microscopy.

Passive immunisation
Inoculation of normal immunoglobulin has a protective effect in people exposed to hepatitis A; there is no immunity for 2 weeks

after inoculation but the immunity thereafter lasts for 4 to 6 months: recommended for anyone travelling to tropical or Mediterranean countries where hepatitis A is endemic and common.

HEPATITIS B

Epidemiology

Hepatitis B is the main cause of post-transfusion hepatitis — now decreasing in incidence as a result of screening blood donations for hepatitis B antigen. Blood may be highly infectious and one extensive epidemic of infection followed the use of yellow fever vaccine during the Second World War which included human serum as a stabilizing agent. Infection can also be spread by the use of communal or inadequately sterilized syringes and needles.

Tattooing and acupuncture: have also been the source of outbreaks of hepatitis B; less obviously, the disease was common amongst *track runners* in Sweden apparently either through communal bathing or by direct inoculation resulting from scratches and minor abrasions caused by running through thickets.

Drug addicts: are at particular risk from hepatitis B; infection is transmitted by sharing of unsterilized syringes used for intravenous administration of drugs.

Sexual transmission: patients attending clinics for sexually-transmitted diseases show a higher incidence of antigen and antibody to the virus than the normal population and the disease is much more common in male homosexuals — and in drug abusers — than in other groups in the community.

Non-parenteral spread: although in many cases a source of parenterally-acquired infection can be discovered, some cases appear to be due to non-parenteral transmission — possibly through close personal contact or sexual intercourse.

Renal dialysis units: Hepatitis B has been a particular problem in renal units: infection is introduced by the blood transfusions required by the patients and spreads from them to other patients and staff. The staff involved has included not only doctors and nurses but also biochemistry and haematology M.L.S.O.s who handle samples of infected blood. There have been several outbreaks of infection, some have been mild with no deaths: in others, like that in

Edinburgh Royal Infirmary in which there was a 30% case fatality rate, the mortality has been high.

Carriers of hepatitis B virus: in Africa and Asia symptomless carriage is common — up to 15% of the population: in Britain the incidence of carriage is about 0.1%. There is increasing evidence that hepatitis B plays a role in primary liver cancer and carriers of the virus show a 300-fold increase in the incidence of this tumour (a common form of cancer in tropical countries).

Acute hepatitis B in pregnancy: is usually followed by infection of the infant; the virus is probably transmitted transplacentally *in utero* or during delivery; the infected babies become chronic carriers of hepatitis B antigen in their blood and around half of them develop persistent hepatitis. Infection of the newborn infant is less common when the mother is a symptomless carrier of hepatitis B virus or antigen; however, more infants become infected in the months after birth presumably due to close contact with their mothers.

Sequelae of hepatitis B: attacks of acute hepatitis B are followed — in around 3% of cases — by the development of *chronic active hepatitis*; this severe disease is associated with liver dysfunction and a fluctuating course leading in many cases to cirrhosis and progressive liver failure. Not all — in fact probably only a minority of — cases of chronic active hepatitis are due to previous hepatitis B.

Chronic persistent hepatitis is a benign and self-limiting disease which may follow hepatitis B; there are mild inflammatory signs in the liver and symptoms are minor or absent; this disease too is probably associated with previous hepatitis B in a minority of patients.

Virology

Hepatitis B antigen is present in the serum of patients in the acute stage of hepatitis B; in most patients the antigen disappears in convalescence but in about 5% of patients the antigen persists for long periods of time.

Electron microscopy: the antigen consists of three types of particle (Fig. 13.1):
1. Spherical particles 22 nm in diameter.
2. Tubular particles 22 nm in diameter.

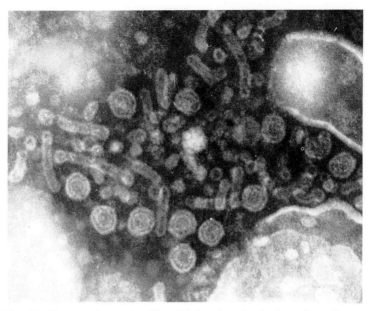

Fig. 13.1 Electron micrographs of hepatitis B antigen showing large 42 nm Dane particles, smaller 22 nm spherical and tubular particles. × 220 000 (Photograph by Dr E.A.C. Follett.)

3. Larger, spherical particles (known as Dane particles) 42 nm in diameter.

Dane particles are the virions of hepatitis B virus, the smaller 22 nm particles being aggregates of coat protein; Dane particles contain circular double-stranded DNA (but this has quite a large single-stranded region) and have a virion-associated DNA-dependent DNA polymerase.

Antigenic structure: Dane particles have the following antigens:
HBsAg: the surface antigen found also on the 22 nm particles.
HBcAg: the antigen of the inner core of the Dane particle.
HBeAg: also associated with the core of the Dane particle and correlated with infectivity.

Antigenic subtypes: the 4 subtypes of hepatitis B antigen are based on HBsAg:

adw

adr

ayw

ayr

All share the group-specific determinant *a* in addition to the allelic *d* and *y* (never found together) and — although less often tested — allelic *w* and *r* (which are also mutually exclusive).

Subtype distribution: the predominant subtype of hepatitis B antigen in various situations is as follows:

Symptomless blood donors	*ad*
Acute hepatitis	*ad* and *ay*
Renal units	*ay*
Drug abuse	*ay*

e antigen: this recently discovered antigen is usually present — although briefly — in patients' blood in the acute phase of hepatitis B; its presence in the blood of cases or carriers correlates with infectivity of the blood. The continuing presence of e antigen also correlates with chronic liver disease and it is found in the blood of a high proportion of patients with chronic active hepatitis following hepatitis B. Conversely: anti-e antibody is usually present in healthy carriers and the infectivity of blood containing it is low.

Antibody to hepatitis B core antigen (HBcAb) appears early in infection whereas *antibody to hepatitis B surface antigen* (HBsAb) appears later during convalescence: antibody to hepatitis B surface antigen is present in about 3 to 9% of the normal population. The incidence is higher in certain groups, e.g. in people with a past history of hepatitis B and hospital staff members.

Diagnosis

Serology
Detection of hepatitis B surface antigen (HBsAg):
  Tests:
1. *Radio-immune assay* — the most sensitive test.
2. *Enzyme immune assay* (EIA): almost as sensitive as radio-immune assay.
3. *Reversed passive haemagglutination*: turkey erythrocytes are coated with hepatitis B antibody prepared in horses; the patient's serum is then tested for haemagglutination with these cells.
4. *Counter immunoelectroosmophoresis* was formerly widely used for detection of hepatitis B antigen. It has been superceded by more sensitive methods of detection.

Detection of e antigen (HBeAg)
1. Radio-immune assay.
Detection of hepatitis B antibody:
1. Radio-immune assay.

Passive immunization: injection of hepatitis B-specific immunoglobulin gives partial but significant protection against the disease: it should be used in people exposed in a single episode involving a high risk of infection e.g. accidental inoculation of blood suspected or known to contain hepatitis B antigen.

Delta agent: is a defective RNA virus found only in the presence of hepatitis B. Hepatitis B virus acts as a keeper in its replication and delta agent contains hepatitis B surface antigen as the outer coat of particle. Found mainly in drug abusers and multiply-transfused patients, its role in disease is uncertain.

Non-A, non B-hepatitis
When it became possible to diagnose both hepatitis A and B in the laboratory, it became clear that there was a third form of hepatitis of which the causal virus was unrelated to either hepatitis A or hepatitis B viruses. Known as non-A, non-B the disease comprises at least three forms of viral hepatitis:

1. Transmitted by blood transfusion or by injection of blood products
2. Sporadic or endemic hepatitis
3. Epidemic water-borne hepatitis

The causal agents appear to be unrelated to each other and to hepatitis A or B.

Widespread epidemics of water-borne non-A, non-B hepatitis have been reported in India. Infection is by the faecal-oral route due to sewage contamination of the water supply. The disease is generally mild except in pregnant women in whom there is a high mortality due to the frequent development of fulminant hepatitis.

14

Antiviral therapy

There is no generally useful therapy for virus infections in any way similar to antibiotic therapy for bacterial disease. However, a few antiviral drugs have been developed which are used mainly for herpesvirus infections.

Note: Viruses are resistant to all antibacterial antibiotics.

Below are some of the principle antiviral drugs:

PURINE AND PYRIMIDINE NUCLEOSIDES
1. Idoxuridine — 5-iodo-2-deoxyuridine
2. Cytarabine — cytosine arabinoside
3. Vidarabine — adenine arabinoside
4. Acyclovir — acycloguanosine

Viruses inhibited: herpesviruses.

Action: inhibit DNA synthesis.

Toxic effects: generally toxic to cells since, with the exception of acyclovir, their action is not specific for viral DNA; acyclovir is phosphorylated by herpes-specific thymidine kinase to monophosphate and it is this form which acts to inhibit virus DNA polymerase; the main side-effects of systemic administration of the nucleosides are bone marrow depression, stomatitis, alopecia, and abnormalities of liver function. Acyclovir has not yet had the necessary large scale trials to determine its side-effects but theoretically these should be much less than with the other compounds.

Indications for use

Herpes keratitis (recurrent dendritic ulcer): local application of 0.1% solution of idoxuridine, preferably every 2 hours, is effective and produces clinical improvement; however, the frequency of recurrences is not reduced.

Skin vesicles due to herpes simplex or varicella-zoster virus may be painful (especially in the case of zoster) or extensive enough to justify therapy. Idoxuridine applied locally produces relief and shortens the duration of pain and lesions. For herpes simplex a 5% solution in dimethyl sulphoxide is usually effective but zoster lesions are best treated with a stronger solution, i.e. 35 or 40% idoxuridine in dimethyl sulphoxide.

Varicella pneumonia: systemic vidarabine administered intravenously is the drug of choice.

Severe varicella or disseminated zoster in immuno-compromised patients: can be effectively treated with intravenous vidarabine; side-effects are usually minimal.

Herpes encephalitis: has also been treated with vidarabine: in one trial this apparently reduced the mortality rate but the efficacy of vidarabine is uncertain. Acyclovir may prove to be better.

Generalised herpes simplex: is a severe disease justifying the use of systemic treatment; cytarabine has been used with success.

Note: acyclovir is the most promising antiherpes drug: it has high activity *in vitro* and should theoretically have little or no effect on host cell DNA. Clinical trials have indicated that it is effective when applied topically in herpes keratitis and intravenously in severe herpes simplex in immunocompromised patients. There were no side-effects. However, further and larger trials are necessary to assess its further role in antiviral chemotherapy.

INTERFERON

Interferon is still by far the more promising antiviral agent: nontoxic, active against all viruses, it may yet prove to be an effective and practicable way of treating and preventing virus infections: unfortunately it has proved impossible to prepare large quantities of human interferon and only small amounts — which are extremely expensive — are available.

Interferon is not a single substance but a family of cellular molecules with regulatory functions which not only inhibit virus replication, but have multiple effects on cell metabolism as well.

There are three main types of human interferon (HuIFN):
1. IFN — α: produced by human leucocytes: formerly known as Le (leucocyte) type I interferon.
2. IFN — β: produced by human fibroblasts: formerly known as F (fibroblast) type I interferon.
3. IFN — γ: produced by human lymphocytes in response to antigenic or mitogenic stimulation: formerly known as IIF (immune) type II interferon.

Interferon for clinical use is produced commercially mainly from leucocytes derived from the buffy coat of blood transfusions: another source of human interferon is the Namalva lymphoblastoid cell line derived from a Burkitt's lymphoma tumour: the quantities of human interferon presently available are very limited and it is therefore used only on an experimental basis. Recently, advances in *genetic engineering* have shown that it is possible to produce interferon using recombinant DNA technology in bacteria. This offers real hope that it will be possible to manufacture large quantities of interferon in the future.

Properties

Cellular protein(s): interferon is a family of cell regulatory molecules released from cells in response to virus infection (and probably to other stimuli also); when interferon is taken up by uninfected cells these become resistant to virus infection; it is produced by cells in tissue culture as well as in intact animals.

Induction: interferon is produced in response to inactivated as well as live viruses; RNA viruses are better inducers than DNA viruses. Synthetic polyribonucleotides are powerful inducers: polyriboinosinic-polyribocytidylic acid (poly rI: poly rC) is a particularly good inducer.

Species-specific: interferon is active only in cells of the same animal species in which it was formed.

Viral susceptibility: all viruses are inhibited by interferon although RNA viruses are generally more susceptible than DNA viruses.

Mode of action: interferon binds to the cell plasma membrane; in cells treated with interferon, viral nucleic acid and protein synthesis are inhibited; adsorption, penetration and uncoating take place normally.

Interferon has two main actions:

(1) *Degradation of mRNA* by an endonuclease which is activated by the oligonucleotide 2, 5 A. The oligonucleotide is itself synthesized by the stimulation of a synthetase activated by the combined effect of interferon and double-stranded RNA.

(2) *Inhibition of protein synthesis*. Interferon and double-stranded RNA also activate a protein kinase which in turn phosphorylates and so inactivates the initiation factor in protein synthesis, eI F-2.

Effect on human virus infections: interferon administered intranasally prevents experimentally-induced rhinovirus infection; it also prevents vaccinia infection if injected intradermally at the site of inoculation. In clinical trials it appears to have an effect — but not a dramatic one — in herpes keratitis, zoster, cytomegalovirus infection, and chronic active hepatitis due to hepatitis B virus.

Effect in cancer: clinical trials with interferon have shown a significant effect in several human tumours such as osteogenic sarcoma, myeloma, lymphoma and breast cancer. Most available supplies of interferon are therefore at present being used for trials in cancer patients.

AMANTADINE (l-adamantine hydrochloride)

Amantadine can prevent influenza A — both naturally-occurring and experimentally-induced; it acts by blocking the penetration of influenza A virus into cells but has no effect on influenza B virus. It is administered orally; side-effects may follow its use — these involve the central nervous system and particularly affect elderly patients; amantadine has never become widely used.

15

Slow virus diseases

Slow virus diseases are diseases with a long incubation period, slow development of symptoms and a protracted, sometimes fatal course. Some are chronic infections with conventional viruses but others are due to unconventional agents which may be viruses but are certainly quite unlike most human pathogenic viruses. Examples of slow virus diseases in man due to conventional viruses are listed in Table 15.1. There are many examples in animals due to a variety of different viruses.

Table 15.1 Slow virus diseases due to conventional viruses

Virus	Disease
Measles	Subacute sclerosing panencephalitis
Rubella	Subacute sclerosing panencephalitis (follows congenital infection)
JC virus, SV_{40}-like virus	Progressive multifocal leuco-encephalopathy.
Hepatitis B	Hepatitis B, chronic active and chronic persistent hepatitis.

Most of the diseases in Table 15.1. have been described in earlier chapters on the appropriate viruses. Progressive multifocal leuco-encephalopathy is described below:

PROGRESSIVE MULTIFOCAL LEUCOENCEPHALOPATHY

This rare disease is now regarded as a slow virus disease due to conventional viruses — in this instance papovaviruses: it is opportunistic in that it is only seen in patients whose health is compromised by pre-existing disease such as leukaemia, reticulosis or immuno-suppressive therapy.

Clinical features

Varied neurological signs: such as hemiparesis, dementia, dysphasia, incoordination, impaired vision and hemianaesthesia.

Duration: usually fatal in 3 to 4 months.

Pathology: multiple foci of demyelination in cerebral haemispheres and cerebellum: brain stem and basal ganglia may also be affected.

Histology: oligodendrocytes with swollen nuclei and intranuclear inclusions are characteristic features.

Virology

Most cases are due to a papovavirus called JC virus or human polyoma virus but some are due to a virus which seems almost identical to SV_{40} — a virus of which monkeys are the natural hosts (see p. 128). JC virus has the following properties:
1. DNA virus with typical papovavirus morphology and containing circular, double-stranded DNA.
2. Grows in human fetal glial tissue cultures; virus growth is recognised by electron microscopy.
3. Haemagglutinates human and guinea pig erythrocytes at 4°C.
4. Infection with the virus is widespread in the community since a considerable proportion of people have antibody to it; there is no evidence that it causes disease in normal people and progressive multifocal leucoencephalopathy is presumably a rare manifestation of infection due to reactivation of latent virus in a compromised host.

SLOW VIRUS DISEASES DUE TO UNCONVENTIONAL AGENTS

There are three slow virus diseases, all of which involve the CNS, and which are due to unconventional agents. These agents are probably viruses but have properties unlike those of other viruses: their structure is unknown and they have never been seen in the electron microscope.

Infections with the agents show the following features:
1. Long incubation period.
2. Protracted, severe, progressive course: virtually always fatal.
3. Pathologically: degeneration of the CNS with status spongiosus.

4. Lesions show no inflammatory reaction.
5. No antibody or other immune response.
   The three slow virus diseases of this type are listed in Table 15.2.

Table 15.2 Slow virus diseases due to unconventional agents.

Virus	Host species	Pathological features	Disease syndrome
Kuru	Man	Subacute cerebellar degeneration; status spongiosus	Postural instability; ataxia, tremor
Creutzfeldt-Jakob disease	Man	Subacute degeneration of brain and spinal cord with status spongiosus of cortex	Presenile dementia; ataxia, spasticity, involuntary movements
Scrapie	Sheep	Subacute cerebellar degeneration	Ataxia, tremor, constant rubbing; susceptibility to infection is genetically determined

SCRAPIE

Scrapie is a neurological disease of sheep common in Britain 200 years ago and now present in sheep in many other countries also. Because of strong evidence that it is due to an infectious agent of the size of a small virus, it has been the subject of a great deal of research.

Clinical features
Natural scrapie affects both sheep and goats; the following are features of natural scrapie in sheep:

Long incubation period: from 2 to 5 years.

Signs and symptoms: affected sheep suffer from excitability, incoordination, ataxia, tremor and continous scratching or rubbing due to sensory neurological disturbance; the symptoms progress to paralysis and death.

Pathology: cerebellar neuronal degeneration with astrocytic proliferation; the status spongiosus found in experimental scrapie is not seen in the natural disease.

Heredity: a major gene controls whether or not sheep develop disease after experimental inoculation; the operation of the gene is complex and depends partly on the strain of agent used for inoculation.

Route of infection: the disease is transmitted by contact in flocks of sheep and probably also vertically from ewes to lambs.

SCRAPIE AGENT

Scrapie can be transmitted by intracerebral or subcutaneous inoculation using the brains of infected sheep. The incubation period varies from 3 to 24 months depending on the strain of agent; the disease can also be transmitted to and passaged in mice with a shorter incubation period of 4 to 8 weeks; experimental infection in mice forms the basic technique of assaying the agent.

Properties of the scrapie agent
1. Small size — 20 to 30 nm.
2. Resistant to ultraviolet-irradiation, formaldehyde and heat (the agent resists 80° for 60 minutes).
3. Does not stimulate antibody production in experimental animals.

No nucleic acid has been demonstrated in the scrapie agent nor has it been seen by electron microscopy; the remarkable resistance to ultraviolet-irradiation suggests that, if nucleic acid is present, it must be in small amounts. Among many theories as to its nature, the most popular at present is that the agent is a viroid like that of potato spindle tuber disease; this is a virus-like agent consisting of a very small piece of RNA protected by nuclear chromatin.

TRANSMISSABLE MINK ENCEPHALOPATHY

A disease due to scrapie agent: mink bred in mink farms have become infected when fed on the heads of scrapie-infected sheep.

KURU

Kuru is a fatal disease found only among the Foré-speaking people in New Guinea. It seems to have appeared about 60 years ago. The incidence increased up until the late 1950s when kuru was responsible for about half the deaths in the Foré-speaking people. The incidence of kuru declined rapidly in the early 1960s.

Clinical features

1. *Kuru* is a native word meaning 'trembling with cold and fever'.
2. *The first or ambulant stage* of the disease starts with unsteadiness in walking, postural instability, ataxia and tremor; facial expressions are poorly controlled and speech becomes slurred and tremulous.
3. *The second or sedentary stage* is reached when the patient cannot walk without support, but can still sit upright unaided.
4. *In the tertiary stage the patient cannot sit upright* without clutching a stick for support; even a gentle push makes the patient lurch violently; the patient becomes progressively more paralysed and emaciated.
5. *Duration* of the disease averages one year but ranges from three months to two years.
6. *Death* is due to bulbar depression or intercurrent infection.
7. *Pathology*: neuronal degeneration in cerebellum with astrocytic hyperplasia, gliosus and status spongiosus; demyelination is minimal or absent.
8. *Sex incidence*: kuru is uncommon in adult males; most patients are women or children of both sexes.
9. *Cannibalism of dead relatives* is thought to have been responsible for the spread of kuru among the Foré people. Men do not usually take part in these cannibalistic feasts. The women and children eat the viscera and brains of relatives including those who have died of kuru. Since these tissues are often inadequately cooked the casual agent may be ingested in active form by those eating brain tissue.
10. *Cannibalism was generally stopped around 1957* and kuru is now declining in incidence: this lends support to the theory that the disease has been spread by cannibalism; on the assumption that kuru is spread in this way, the *incubation period* appears to be from 4 to 20 years.

Causal agent

Transmission experiments: intracerebral inoculation of brain tissue from kuru victims into chimpanzees and other monkeys causes the animals to develop the symptoms of kuru after an incubation period of two years. After passage, the incubation period is shortened to about one year.

The reproduction of the disease in experimental animals is strong evidence that kuru is due to an infectious agent. However, attempts to cultivate the causal agent from both human and chimpanzee tissues in tissue cultures have been unsuccessful.

Experimental studies in chimpanzees have shown that the agent has the following properties:

1. *Passes filters* of 100 nm pore diameter — indicating that it is in the size range of viruses.
2. *Present in infected brain tissue* to a titre of 10^6 infectious units per ml.
3. *Present in spleen, liver and kidney* of infected animals although the organs appear normal.
4. *Can be transmitted peripherally* (i.e. by combined intravenous, subcutaneous, intramuscular and intraperitoneal routes) as well as intracerebrally.
5. *No antibody* to the agent has been detected in either humans or chimpanzees with kuru.

CREUTZFELDT-JAKOB DISEASE

A rare progressive neurological disease characterized by a combination of presenile dementia with symptoms due to lesions in the spinal cord.

Clinical features

1. *Prodromal stage*: the disease starts with tiredness, apathy and vague neurological symptoms.
2. *Second stage*: the patient develops ataxia, dysarthria and progressive spasticity of the limbs, this is associated with dementia and often involuntary movements such as myoclonic jerks or choreoathetoid movements.
3. *The disease progresses steadily* until death — usually from about six months to two years after the onset of symptoms.
4. *Pathology*: diffuse atrophy with status spongiosus in the cerebral cortex; atrophy also in basal ganglia, cerebellum, substantia nigra and anterior horn cells.

Causal agent

Transmission experiments: the disease is reproduced in chimpanzees and other monkeys after intracerebral inoculation of brain tissue from cases of the disease; the incubation period is from 11 to 14 months; the disease can also be transmitted peripherally (by combined intravenous, intraperitoneal and intramuscular routes).

Human infection: the natural route of infection is unknown but Creutzfeldt-Jakob disease has been accidentally transmitted via a corneal graft to the recipient. Transmission has also been reported via electrodes used for electro-encephalography from a patient with the disease to other patients in whom the electrodes were subsequently implanted.

Spiroplasma: have been reported in the brain of patients with Creutzfeldt-Jakob disease: These are spiral or helical mycoplasma: further confirmation of this observation is required before an association with the disease can be assumed.

Note: slow virus diseases due to unconventional agents are attracting considerable interest because of the possibility that certain human neurological diseases of unknown cause (e.g. multiple sclerosis, amyotrophic lateral sclerosis, Altzheimer's disease) might be due to similar agents.

16

Tumour viruses

Many viruses cause cancer in animals. So far no virus has been shown to cause cancer in man.

The oncogenic or tumour-producing properties of a virus can be shown in two ways:
1. Inoculation of the virus into experimental animals produces tumours;
2. The virus transforms normal cells in tissue culture into cells with characteristics of malignant or cancer cells.

Note: tumour viruses include both RNA and DNA viruses.

Transformation of cells in tissue culture
Transformation of cells in tissue culture is believed to be analogous to the induction by viruses of cancer in intact animals. Transformed cells show several altered properties when compared to normal transformed cells.

1. Morphological change
Transformed cells are first detected as foci of cells which are different in appearance from the background of normal untransformed cells.

2. Loss of contact inhibition
Normal cells are inhibited from dividing when they grow out to form a monolayer and come in contact with each other. This is called contact or topo-inhibition. Transformed cells do not show this and continue to divide on contact so that they grow in a criss-cross pattern and pile up on one another.

3. Low serum requirement
Transformed cells can grow and divide in medium with a low concentration of serum. Normal cells are inhibited from dividing unless a high concentration of serum is present.

4. Increased agglutinability with plant lectins
Transformed cells agglutinate in high dilutions of plant lectins such as concanavelin A and wheat germ agglutinin. Normal cells agglutinate only in low dilutions of lectins.

5. Growth in agar
Transformed cells are able to divide and form colonies when suspended in semi-solid agar or methylcellulose. Normal cells are unable to grow under these conditions.

6. New antigens
New antigens can be demonstrated in transformed cells which are not present in normal cells. These include the *T or tumour antigen* found in the nucleus which is an early non-structural virus protein made briefly during virus replication but constantly present in transformed cells. The TSTA or *tumour-specific transplantation antigen* is a surface antigen responsible for the graft rejection reaction when animals are inoculated with transformed tumour cells. Animals immunized against this antigen reject tumour cell grafts.

7. Transplantability
Transformed cells show increased transplantability compared to normal cells in that they show an enhanced ability to produce tumours on inoculation into animals.

8. Integrated viral DNA
The most important feature of transformed cells is that they contain a fragment of viral DNA integrated into the DNA of the cell chromosome. This DNA functions and its gene products are responsible for maintaining the transformed state and for expressing the various virus functions (e.g. T antigens) detected in transformed cells.

RNA TUMOUR VIRUSES

RNA tumour viruses cause natural cancer in the host animal. They also produce tumours on inoculation into experimental animals. Although the sarcoma viruses transform cells most of the leukaemia viruses do not.

Morphology
RNA tumour viruses now classified as retroviruses have two types of particle:

1. *C-type particles*. Most RNA tumour viruses have spherical enveloped particles surrounded by spikes or knobs and containing a central core which is composed of RNA and protein (Fig. 16.1).

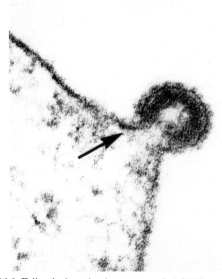

Fig. 16.1 Feline leukaemia virus — a typical RNA tumour virus particle budding through the plasma membrane on its release from the cell. The continuity between the cell surface membrane and the virion is indicated by the arrow and the spikes on the surface of the outer virion membrane are clearly seen. x 190 000 (Photograph by Dr Helen Laird).

2. *B-type particles*. Mouse mammary tumour virus has particles similar to C-type particles but with an eccentric core or nucleoid.

   All RNA tumour virus particles contain the enzyme reverse transcriptase (see Chapter 2).

Genome structure

The genome of RNA tumour viruses contains four genes:

1. The *gag* gene which codes for the core protein antigens of the virus particle. These are cleaved from a larger precursor protein.
2. The *pol* gene which codes for the protein that is the reverse transcriptase.
3. The *env* gene which codes for the glycoprotein envelope proteins of the virion.
4. The *onc* gene which is responsible for transformation.

Transformation

The *onc* gene of RNA tumour viruses codes for a *protein kinase* which is responsible for transformation. This enzyme phosphorylates tyrosine residues and probably affects cell regulation and so produces malignant transformation of cells (see also Chapter 2). The *onc* gene seems to be a cellular gene acquired by the virus RNA genome: its activity is probably controlled by a virus-coded promoter produced by terminal repeated sequences in the virus genome.

Epidemiology

Most animal species in which a detailed search has been made have been shown to harbour RNA tumour viruses. Man is an exception to this and extensive research has so far failed to reveal an undoubted human RNA tumour virus.

Transmission

Transmission of RNA tumour viruses from animal to animal takes place in three ways:

1. *Horizontal*: in which the virus spreads by direct contact between infected and susceptible animals. This is an important route of infection in naturally-occurring infection in outbred animals not reared in a laboratory such as cats.
2. *Congenital*: a form of vertical transmission in which the virus spreads from mother to offspring either by infection *in utero* or via the mother's milk.
3. *Genetic*: Another form of vertical transmission but in this case the virus is inherited in the form of a *provirus* or viral DNA transcript integrated into the chromosomes of the germ cells of the parent animal. The viruses produced from proviruses are known as *endogenous* viruses and are typical RNA tumour viruses: however, although some are tumour-producing on inoculation into experimental animals many are not. Endogenous RNA viruses are usually present in a repressed state but can be induced by various agents so that their genes are derepressed with consequent production of the virus in the animal.

Endogenous RNA viruses are known to be present in a repressed state in normal cells of chickens, mice, cats and baboons.

Oncogene theory

The oncogene theory states that normal cellular chromosomes contain two sets of genes: one, the *virogene*, codes for an endogenous RNA virus, the second, the *oncogene*, is a transforming or tumour-producing gene which when derepressed causes tumour formation in the animal. When both are derepressed together the animal produces the RNA virus and develops cancer. Sometimes one gene only may be derepressed causing either RNA virus production without cancer or cancer without RNA virus replication.

TUMOURS PRODUCED BY RNA TUMOUR VIRUSES

Most RNA tumour viruses can be classified as:
1. Sarcoma viruses.
2. Leukaemia viruses.

Sarcoma viruses

Sarcoma viruses readily transform cells in tissue culture and produce solid tumours — fibrosarcomas — on inoculation into animals of the host species. Most are defective so that, in order to replicate, they require the presence of a helper virus (usually a leukaemia virus of the same species) to supply the product of the defective gene. The defective gene is the *env* gene and as a result sarcoma viruses have the same type-specific neutralising antigen in their envelope as the helper leukaemia virus.

Leukaemia viruses

Leukaemia viruses produce leukaemia on inoculation into animals. Many do not transform cells in tissue culture although some do so. Leukaemia viruses are not defective and generally replicate well in tissue culture. They do not produce CPE and cell growth and division are not affected.

Table 16.1 lists the principle RNA tumour viruses, their host animal species and the tumours produced.

Table 16.1   RNA tumour viruses

Host animal	Virus	Tumour
Chickens	Rous sarcoma virus	Sarcoma in chickens
	Avian leukosis viruses	Fowl leukaemia
Mice	Mouse sarcoma virus	Sarcoma in mice
	Mouse leukaemia viruses	Mouse leukaemia
	Mouse mammary tumour virus	Breast cancer in mice
Cats	Feline sarcoma virus	Sarcoma in cats
	Feline leukaemia virus	Cat leukaemia
Primates	Simian sarcoma virus	Sarcoma in marmosets
	Gibbon ape leukaemia virus	Leukaemia in gibbon apes

The following are brief descriptions of some of the best-studied RNA tumour viruses.

1. *Rous sarcoma virus*: discovered by Peyton Rous in 1911 who found that the cell-free filtrate from fowl tumours produced sarcomas when injected into fowls; the virus can be assayed *in vitro* by the production of tumour-like foci due to transformation in monolayers of chick embryo fibroblasts.

   Rous sarcoma virus can produce tumours in rabbits, mice, guinea-pigs, hamsters and monkeys in addition to fowls.

2. *Avian leukosis viruses*: infection with these viruses is widespread in poultry flocks — often without causing tumours. Occasionally lymphomatosis — a kind of leukaemia in fowls — becomes epidemic and kills up to half the stock of poultry farms. In the natural state, leukosis viruses are often transmitted 'vertically', i.e. from hen to chick; chicks are infected in the egg and contamination of eggs — including domestic hen eggs — is frequent. Uninfected and non-immune chicks are susceptible to 'horizontal' transmission of infection from fowls which excrete the virus

3. *Mouse leukaemia viruses*: these viruses were isolated from laboratory bred mouse strains and produce leukaemia on inoculation into newborn mice; after passage through susceptible animals in the laboratory, their potency becomes increased and they can produce leukaemia in adult mice — and sometimes in rats and hamsters also. Laboratory mice vary in the incidence of naturally-occurring leukaemia; when low leukaemic mice are inoculated with mouse leukaemia virus, their offspring show a high incidence of leukaemia; the virus can therefore be transmitted vertically.

4. *Mouse sarcoma viruses*: defective, serologically related to mouse leukaemia viruses (see above); produce solid tumours and resemble Rous sarcoma virus in many properties.

5. *Mouse mammary tumour virus — formerly called Bittner virus*: this virus is transmitted in the milk of mother mice to their offspring; female offspring of infected mothers show a high incidence (92%) of breast cancer but if fostered by normal mothers the incidence of breast cancer in the offspring is 8%.

   Tumour development by mouse mammary tumour virus depends on three different factors:

   a. The presence of the virus

   b. Hormonal influences: hormones are required to stimulate

mammary tissue and render it susceptible to tumour development.

   c. Genetic factors: strains of mice vary in their susceptibility to the induction of mammary cancer.

6. *Feline leukaemia virus*: cats are randomly bred and have not been subjected to the intensive in-breeding of most laboratory strains of chickens and mice; feline leukaemia virus spreads in the natural state by horizontal transmission and there have been several reports of clusters of leukaemia in domestic cats (a cluster is one household in which several cats have developed leukaemia suggesting that the disease is due to infection). Infection with feline leukaemia virus, detected by antibody studies, is much more common in urban stray cats than in domestic pets or rural stray cats. Not all infected cats develop leukaemia — in fact leukaemia is a relatively rare consequence of infection.

DNA TUMOUR VIRUSES

DNA tumour viruses
DNA tumour viruses are easier to study in the laboratory than RNA tumour viruses but have one great disadvantage: most do not cause naturally-occurring cancer in the host animal. Nevertheless they are highly oncogenic on inoculation into laboratory animals and efficently transform cells in tissue culture; they are therefore excellent model systems in which to investigate the molecular basis of viral carcinogenesis.

Replication
In permissive cells (i.e. cells in which they can grow) DNA tumour viruses replicate and cause CPE in much the same way as non-oncogenic viruses; however, they stimulate cellular DNA synthesis instead of switching it off as non-tumour viruses do.

Transformation
DNA viruses transform non-permissive cells in which they cannot replicate; cells transformed by DNA viruses do not shed virus like RNA virus-transformed cells. Although in some cases the whole DNA virus genome is integrated into the host cell chromosome, in others only a small fragment of virus DNA is present.

   Table 16.2 lists the principal DNA tumour viruses with the host animal and the tumours they cause.

Table 16.2   DNA tumour viruses

Host	Virus	Tumour
Mice	Polyoma virus	Multiple primary tumours in hamsters
Monkeys	Simian virus 40(SV$_{40}$)	Sarcomas in hamsters
Man	Adenoviruses	Sarcomas in hamsters
Chickens	Marek's disease virus (a herpesvirus)	Malignant neurolymphomatosis

1. *Polyoma virus*: polyoma virus is endemic in mouse colonies but does not cause naturally-occurring cancer in mice. The virus haemagglutinates guinea-pig erythrocytes and can be assayed by plaque formation in mouse embryo tissue cultures; it is therefore relatively easy to study in the laboratory; it transforms hamster cells in tissue culture into cells with the properties of malignant or cancer cells.
2. *SV$_{40}$ or simian virus 40*: a common contaminant of monkey kidney tissue cultures; it either produces no CPE or sometimes vacuolation of the cells and is often present in monkey kidneys as a latent virus. SV$_{40}$ causes tumours on injection into hamsters and transforms cells — including human cells — in tissue culture. The main importance of SV$_{40}$ is that it is a highly oncogenic virus. It was a common contaminant of early batches of poliovaccine; as a result, thousands of young children were accidentally inoculated with the virus but apparently without ill-effect.
3. *Adenoviruses*: commonly cause respiratory infections in man but many types cause tumours on inoculation into hamsters; types 12, 18 and 31 are the most highly oncogenic.
   Adenovirus DNA can form 'hybrids' with SV$_{40}$ DNA; the nucleic acid of the hybrid contains fragments of the genomes of both viruses; hybrids are enclosed in protein coats specified by the adenovirus; cells transformed by the hybrids contain SV$_{40}$-specific antigens showing persistence of part of the SV$_{40}$ genome.
4. *Marek's disease virus*: causes a cancerous disease in chickens affecting both neural and lymphoid tissues; it spreads horizontally from bird to bird in the flock, being shed from the feather follicles of infected birds. The virus does not transform cells in tissue culture although it replicates well in tissue culture; Marek's disease virus is one of the few DNA tumour viruses

which causes naturally occurring cancer in the host species. Epidemics of Marek's disease are a commercial problem in flocks; a vaccine prepared against Marek's disease virus gives good protection against the disease.

WARTS

Warts are common infections of most animal species. Warts are non-malignant tumours of the skin characterized by marked proliferation of epithelial cells. Most regress spontaneously but warts are notoriously difficult to treat. Certain types of wart occasionally become cancerous but most are entirely benign.

Papillomaviruses: Warts are due to papillomaviruses which are specific for the various animal species which are their natural host. Papillomaviruses are members of the papovavirus family to which polyoma virus and SV_{40} virus also belong.

HUMAN WARTS

Clinical features
Warts can be divided into four categories depending on their clinical appearance and site:
1. *Skin*: especially of the hands and feet (plantar warts): plantar warts sometimes become epidemic in children as a result of cross-infection acquired in swimming baths. Skin warts never undergo malignant change.
2. *Genital* (*condylomata acuminata*): usually transmitted by sexual intercourse, genital warts sometimes become very large. Rarely, they undergo cancerous change.
3. *Oral*: warts on the buccal mucosa are rare in Britain but not uncommon in American Indians and Eskimos.
4. *Laryngeal papillomas* are also rare in Britain but are common in Southern USA. Most often seen in children and sometimes in infants due to infection acquired at birth from genital warts in the mother. Laryngeal papillomas do not become malignant but they tend to recur causing progressive damage to the vocal cords.

Virology
1. Papillomaviruses are papovaviruses and contain double-stranded circular DNA.

2. Typical papovavirus morphology on electron microscopy (Fig.16.2) but larger (50 nm) than polyoma or SV_{40} viruses (40 nm).
3. Cannot be cultivated *in vitro* or *in vivo* (i.e. in experimental laboratory animals).
4. Different types of human wart virus can be distinguished by biochemical techniques (restriction enzyme DNA analysis, DNA hybridization). There is a marked tendency for certain clinical kinds of wart to be associated with particular types of virus.

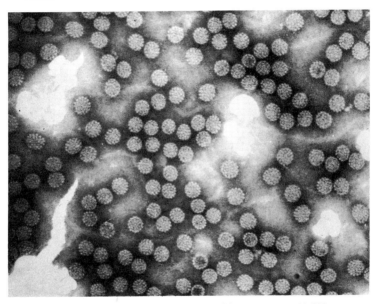

Fig. 16.2 Wart virus. The virus particles have cubic symmetry. × 90 000. (Photograph by Dr E.A.C. Follett.)

Shope papilloma virus is of unusual interest: it is the cause of papillomas in wild rabbits and is normally spread by insect vectors; papillomas are produced when the virus is inoculated into wild rabbits and in these tumours cancerous change is relatively rare. In domestic rabbits, Shope papilloma virus produces a higher incidence of papillomas and cancerous changes are observed far more often. Virus cannot be cultured from the tumours which have undergone cancerous change.

VIRUSES AND HUMAN CANCER

Considerable research effort is being devoted to the investigation of

the role of viruses in human cancer; the main interest at present is in three fields of research:
1. EB virus and Burkitt's lymphoma.
2. Type 2 herpes simplex and cancer of the cervix.
3. RNA tumour viruses and various human tumours.

1. EB virus and Burkitt's lymphoma

Burkitt's lymphoma is a highly malignant tumour which is common in African children. It is primarily a tumour of lymphoid tissue but the earliest manifestations of disease are large tumours of the jaw and, in girls, sometimes of the ovaries; it spreads rapidly with widespread metastases. Burkitt's lymphoma is very sensitive to cytotoxic drugs and excellent results, with long-term remissions and possibly even cures, have been described in patients treated with this form of chemotherapy.

There is a striking *geographical distribution*: the incidence of the tumour in Africa is almost completely confined to areas with altitude and minimum annual temperature and rainfall which correspond to areas in which disease-carrying insect vectors are found. It has therefore been suggested that Burkitt's lymphoma may be due to a virus spread by an insect vector. Occasional cases have also been reported outside Africa, e.g. in Western Europe and the USA.

EB virus is probably the cause of Burkitt's lymphoma; the virus was first found in cultures of cells established from Burkitt's lymphoma and virus DNA is present in the lymphoblasts of the tumour. Patients with Burkitt's lymphoma uniformly have antibody to the virus — detected by the fluorescent antibody technique although so also do a considerable proportion of healthy adults; it is therefore clear that infection with EB virus *per se* does not cause Burkitt's lymphoma.

It has been suggested that the geographical distribution of the disease may be due to the fact that the areas where Burkitt's lymphoma is found are also those areas in which the population are virtually all heavily infected with *malaria*. In these circumstances the reticulo-endothelial system is heavily infiltrated with malarial parasites and this may cause an abnormal response to infection with EB virus. As a result, EB virus, instead of producing symptomless infection or a benign proliferation of lymphoid tissue (as in infectious mononucleosis) becomes frankly oncogenic and causes cancerous change in lymphoid tissue (as in Burkitt's lymphoma).

Nasopharyngeal carcinoma: is a tumour which shows a striking racial or genetic incidence. For example, it is particularly common among the Southern Chinese. Nasopharyngeal carcinoma also seems to be associated with EB virus and virus DNA is regularly present in the malignant epithelial cells of the tumour.

2. Type 2 herpes simplex virus and cancer of the cervix

Women with cervical cancer have a higher incidence of antibodies to type 2 herpes simplex virus than comparable groups of matched control women. Type 2 herpes simplex virus does not produce tumours when inoculated into experimental rodents but it transforms rodent embryo cells in tissue culture and the transformed cells cause tumours on inoculation into experimental animals. The type 2 virus genome has been shown to become integrated into the chromosomes of the transformed cells. Type 2 herpes simplex messenger RNA and proteins have been reported to be present in cervical cancer tissue.

3. RNA tumour viruses and human cancer

The large number of RNA tumour viruses which have been isolated from animals including primates, many of which cause natural cancer in the host species, is the chief reason for suspecting that a human RNA tumour virus may exist which is responsible for some forms of cancer. Recently, a new virus of this type, unrelated to any of the animal RNA tumour viruses has been isolated from cases of T-cell leukaemia/lymphoma — a rare human cancer. Antibody to an internal structural protein of the virus has been demonstrated in some of the patients.

17

Chlamydial diseases

Chlamydiae are widespread in human and animal populations. They are not viruses although, by tradition, they are usually handled in virus laboratories. They are really bacteria but differ from bacteria in being unable to grow on inanimate media. Below are some of their laboratory properties.

Bacteriology of chlamydiae
1. Contain both DNA and RNA.
2. Larger than most viruses, 250–500 nm: visible by light microscopy.
3. Replicate only within living cells: the growth cycle is complex and includes a stage of binary fusion.
4. Grow in tissue culture: best cultivated in McCoy or HeLa 229 cells treated with cycloheximide or idoxuridine to stop cell division: chlamydial growth is recognised by the development of intracytoplasmic inclusions detected by Giemsa staining.
5. Grow in yolk sac of chick embryos.
6. Sensitive to tetracycline, erythromycin, sulphonamides.

Table 17.1 shows a classification of chlamydiae with some of their properties.

Table 17.1 Chlamydiae

Subgroup	Hosts	Main diseases	Serotypes
A *Chlamydia trachomatis*	Man	Oculogenital	D, E, F, G, H, I, J, K.
		Trachoma	A, B, C.
		Lymphogranuloma venereum	1, 2, 3.
B *Chlamydia psittaci*	Various animals (including birds)	Psittacosis	—

CHLAMYDIA TRACHOMATIS

C. trachomatis is widespread as a genital infection in human populations and is generally transmitted by sexual intercourse. Infection in women is usually symptomless but, in men, it is responsible for about half the cases of non-specific genital infection. It also causes eye disease, pneumonia, and lymphogranuloma venereum.

1. **Non-specific genital infection**
   Also known as non-specific urethritis and by far the commonest sexually-transmitted disease in Britain: its incidence is continuing to rise.
   Clinical features: acute urethritis with urethral discharge, frequency, dysuria: there may be cystitis, epididymitis and prostatitis — or proctatitis in homosexual males. Reiter's syndrome (a triad of urethritis, arthritis and conjunctivitis is seen in a small proportion (less than 1%) of cases. Female infection commonly involves the cervix: although the cervicitis is sometimes accompanied by mild vaginitis with discharge, it is usually symptomless.
   Treatment: Tetracycline — but relapses are frequent.

2. **Ocular infection**
   C. trachomatis causes three types of eye infection:
   (i) Neonatal ophthalmia
   (ii) Inclusion conjunctivitis
   (iii) Trachoma.
   Neonatal ophthalmia and inclusion conjunctivitis are seen in countries with temperate climates like Britain: trachoma is a disease of tropical countries.
   (i) *Neonatal ophthalmia* (also called inclusion blennorrhoea).
   Seen in babies born to mothers with cervicitis as a result of contamination acquired during passage through the infected birth canal.
   Clinically: a mucopurulent conjunctivitis appearing 4–14 days after birth.
   Treatment: topical application of tetracycline.
   (ii) *Inclusion conjunctivitis*
   A disease mainly of children but sometimes of adults also. Probably acquired by indirect contact from genital infection: for example, outbreaks have been reported where infection has spread amongst children at swimming baths (swimming pool conjunctivitis).
   Clinically: a follicular conjunctivitis with mucopurulent discharge: chlamydial eye infection sometimes results in

punctate keratitis in which there is corneal involvement.
Treatment: topical application of tetracycline.
(iii) *Trachoma*
A major cause of blindness in the world and a scourge of tropical countries: a tragic disease — especially as it responds well to treatment: spread is from case to case by contact, contaminated fomites and flies.
Clinically: a severe follicular conjunctivits with pannus (i.e. invasion of the cornea by blood vessels): corneal scarring which results in blindness is a common sequel.
Treatment: topical application of tetracycline.

3. Pneumonia
Now a recognised complication of chlamydial infection in neonates. Although conjunctivitis is a more common manifestation, pneumonia is seen in about a fifth of infected infants.
Clinically: often preceded by upper respiratory tract symptoms: the pneumonia is relatively mild with dry spasmodic cough and rapid breathing: the infants are not usually febrile. Chest X-rays show diffuse infiltration of the lungs.
Treatment: erythromycin.

4. Lymphogranuloma venereum
A disease which is common in tropical countries but almost unknown in temperate climates. Cases in Britain are rare and the infection has almost invariably been acquired abroad: the disease is generally sexually-transmitted.
Clinical features: in males, the primary lesion is a painless ulcer on the penis which is often unnoticed. The disease then takes the form of the inguinal syndrome in which there is painful enlargement of the inguinal and femoral lymph nodes which later may suppurate to form buboes. The *genito-anorectal syndrome* is the most common disease in women: infection involves the vagina and cervix — usually without symptoms — but the infection can then spread via the lymphatics to the rectum causing proctatitis with bleeding and purulent discharge from the anus.
Treatment: Sulphonamides or tetracycline.

Diagnosis

Isolation

Specimens: genital, eye swabs; sputum.

Culture: in McCoy cells treated with cycloheximide (or idoxuridine) to prevent cell division: HeLa 229 cells can also be used.

Observe: for typical intracytoplasmic inclusions by a modified Giemsa stain.

Direct demonstration

Specimens: smears from lesions.

Examine: for specific immunofluorescence or typical intracytoplasmic inclusions

Serology
1. *Immunofluorescence tests* are type-specific so that sera must be tested against the appropriate range of serotypes (i.e. D, E, F, G, H, I, J, K for most chlamydial infections in Britain).
   IgM tests for the presence of IgM antibody are increasingly used in diagnosis as an indicator of recent infection: detected by type-specific immunofluorescent test.
2. *Complement fixation tests*: still widely used although less sensitive than immunofluorescent tests. Chlamydiae share a common group complement fixing antigen so that it is only necessary to use one strain as antigen.

Chlamydia psittaci
Chlamydia of sub-group B infect a wide variety of animals. The most dangerous from the point of view of human infection are chlamydial infections in birds. Infected birds often, but not always, show signs of disease and this is known as *ornithosis*. When the birds belong to the psittacine family (e.g. budgerigars and parrots) the disease is known as *psittacosis*. The human disease is also called psittacosis — even if it has been acquired from non-psittacine birds: however the majority of human cases are, in fact, acquired from pet budgerigars or parrots.

In Britain, psittacosis is a rare disease although the incidence has risen sharply over the past two years. Outbreaks of infection involving veterinary surgeons and workers in processing plants have been traced to infected flocks of ducks.

Psittacosis

Clinically: Psittacosis most often takes the form of a *primary atypical pneumonia*: the patients have fever, cough and dyspnoea with extensive opacities in the lung fields on chest X-ray. Males are affected more often than females. The disease ranges in severity from a mild influenza-like illness to a severe disease with generalised toxaemic features. Psitticosis is sometimes fatal although the case fatality rate is low (probably less than 1%). Rarely, psittacosis may cause infective endocarditis, as well as myocarditis and pericarditis: renal involvement and disseminated intravascular coagulation are occasional complications.

Treatment: tetracycline

Diagnosis:

Serology
Complement fixation test: using the chlamydial common group antigen.

18

Rickettsial diseases

Rickettsiae are not viruses — in fact they are like bacteria in their properties. Traditionally, however, they are diagnosed in virus laboratories.

There are two kinds of rickettsiae:
(1) Rickettsiae
(2) Coxiellae.

The main difference between them is that coxiellae are resistant to drying.

RICKETTSIAE

Rickettsial diseases are world-wide in distribution but are not found in Britain. The main diseases are listed in Table 18.1.

CLINICAL FEATURES

Acute febrile illness with rash: the rash is usually maculopapular, occasionally vesicular. Rickettsial infections are generally severe diseases: haemorrhagic complications and lymphadenopathy are common.

Fatality rate: is often high in untreated cases (e.g. up to 20% with certain rickettsiae): with antibiotic treatment, the mortality is low.

Recurrent infection (Brill-Zinsser disease) is seen with typhus: recrudences may be years after the primary illness and are usually mild.

Treatment: tetracycline or chloramphenicol.

Vectors: rickettsiae are transmitted to man via infected arthropods, e.g. ticks, lice, and fleas. There is no human case-to-case transmis-

Table 18.1 Rickettsial diseases

	Typhus group		Spotted fever group	Tsutsugamushi group
	Typhus	Murine typhus	Rocky Mountain fever; other tickborne fevers	Scrub typhus (tsutsugamushi fever)
Disease				
Geographical distribution	America, Balkans, East Europe, Asia, Africa	World-wide	USA, Canada, Central, South America	Far East
Causal organism	*R. prowazeki*	*R. typhi*	*R. rickettsi*	*R. tsutsugamushi*
Vector	Louse	Flea	Tick	Mite
Reservoir	Man, flying squirrels (USA)	Rats	Ticks, sometimes rodents	Mites, possibly wild rodents
Weil-Felix reaction				
Proteus OX:19	+	+	+★	–
Proteus OX:K	–	–	–	+
Proteus OX:2	±	±	+★	–

★ Variable.

sion. Arthropods infect man by biting or by contamination of skin scratches with infected faeces (e.g. in typhus and murine typhus).

Reservoirs: usually small animals, e.g. rodents, sometimes the vectors themselves (Table 18.1).

Proteus: rickettsiae share 0 antigens with certain *Proteus* species. Rickettsial disease can be diagnosed by detecting raised antibody titres in agglutination tests with appropriate *Proteus* strains: known as the Weil-Felix reaction (Table 18.1).

Bacteriology
1. Large (relative to viruses) coccobacilli approximately 300 nm in diameter.
2. Can be seen by light microscope with Giemsa or Macchiavello's stain, the organisms staining purplish and red respectively.
3. Contain both DNA and RNA (unlike viruses).
4. Replicate intracellularly but by binary fission: best isolated in guinea pigs or mice.
5. Rapidly killed by drying.
6. Sensitive to chloramphenicol and tetracycline.

Diagnosis

Serology
(1) *Complement fixation test* ⎫
(2) *Weil-Felix reaction*   ⎬   Detect group-specific antibody
(3) *Immunofluorescence* ⎭
(4) *Toxin neutralization*: detection of antibody by testing for the protective effect of patient's serum on a lethal dose of rickettsiae inoculated into mice: a highly specific test that can identify the species of rickettsiae causing infection.

Isolation

Scrub typhus: can be diagnosed by isolation of *R. tsutsugamushi* in mice.

Control
Vaccines are available for typhus and Rocky Mountain Spotted Fever. Control of vectors may cut short an epidemic.

Q FEVER

Coxiella burneti is distributed world-wide — including Britain. It is common in domestic animals and causes Q or 'query' fever. Although this is a sporadic disease in Britain, it was first described as an outbreak of respiratory disease amongst meat workers in Queensland, Australia.

Clinical features

Signs and symptoms: classically those of a pyrexia of unknown origin (PUO): headache (a prominent symptom) with fever, generalized aches and anorexia; the pulse is slow and a proportion of cases have enlargement of the liver with abnormal liver function tests; more rarely, there may be splenomegaly; Q fever is a generalized septicaemic infection.

Pneumonia: about half of the patients have the signs and symptoms of primary atypical pneumonia with patchy consolidation of the lungs on chest X-ray.

Duration: about 2 weeks but the course is sometimes prolonged for 4 or more weeks especially in patients over 40 years old.

Prognosis: is good and complete recovery is usual.

Infective endocarditis: rarely Q fever may be followed by chronic infection with involvement of the heart valves and formation of vegetations. The signs and symptoms are similar to those of bacterial infective endocarditis i.e. fever, finger clubbing, anaemia, heart murmurs and splenomegaly. Liver enlargement is common; the disease is seen in patients in whom the heart valves are damaged by rheumatic heart disease or congenital malformation; unlike Q fever, the prognosis in Q fever endocarditis is poor.

Treatment

Q fever can be successfully treated with tetracycline or chloramphenicol.

Endocarditis: requires long-term treatment with tetracycline; this tends to suppress rather than eradicate the organism and careful follow-up is necessary; replacement of the diseased heart valves by valve prostheses may be life-saving if there is severe cardiac failure. Even with long-term antibiotic therapy there is a relatively high mortality rate although, recently, there have been encouraging reports of long-term survival in several cases of the disease.

Epidemiology

Animal reservoirs: infection is endemic in domestic sheep and cattle; ticks are also often infected and probably play a role in spreading *C. burneti* amongst animals.

Geographical distribution: the disease is world-wide.

Route of human infection: mainly by handling infected animals or by inhalation of contaminated dust; placentas of infected animals are heavily contaminated; infection may also be spread by drinking unpasteurized contaminated milk from infected cows.

Occupational hazard: workers who handle animals have an increased risk of Q fever but, even in them, the disease is relatively rare.

Sex incidence: the majority of patients are male — probably reflecting the occupational hazard.

Seasonal incidence: Q fever is more common in spring and the early summer months.

Bacteriology

C. burneti is similar to the rickettsiae in its properties but differs in being resistant to drying; it can be cultivated in the yolk sac of the chick embryo and infects laboratory animals e.g. guinea pigs.

Diagnosis

Serology

Complement fixation test: with two different preparations of *C. burneti* as antigens:

1. *Phase 1 antigen*: freshly isolated strains of *C. burneti* give no reaction with sera of acute cases but react well with sera from patients with long-standing chronic infection (i.e. endocarditis).
2. *Phase 2 antigen*: strains of *C. burneti* after repeated passage in or adaptation to eggs, react well with sera of acute cases as well as sera from long-standing infections.

Acute Q fever

Serology: complement fixation test with phase 2 antigen.

Q fever endocarditis

Serology: complement fixation test with both phase 1 and phase 2 antigens: patients have high — usually very high — titres of antibodies to both antigens.

Direct demonstration of *C. burneti* in smears of vegetations on heart valves (taken at post-mortem) and stained with Macchiavello's stain: *C. burneti* is detected as minute red cocco-bacilli.

Isolation: by inoculation of guinea pigs with material from valvular vegetations and spleen: after an interval the guinea pig sera are tested for antibodies to *C. burneti* by complement fixation test.

19

Mycoplasma pneumoniae

Mycoplasma pneumoniae is a bacterium, not a virus, but is unusual in that it lacks the peptidoglycan cell wall characteristic of bacteria. For historical reasons *M. pneumoniae* infection is usually diagnosed in virus laboratories mainly because the principal disease it causes was for a long time regarded as 'virus pneumonia'.

CLINICAL FEATURES

Respiratory infections

M. pneumoniae is primarily a respiratory pathogen. Although many, probably most, of the infections it causes are mild or even symptomless, it is an important cause of lower respiratory disease.

1. Primary atypical pneumonia

Formerly known as 'virus pneumonia', with symptoms of fever, hacking non-productive cough and often a severe headache: marked weakness and tiredness are common. On X-ray, there is patchy consolidation of the lungs. On average the disease lasts for about ten days but in a proportion of cases symptoms persist for considerably longer.

Note

Primary atypical pneumonia is also caused — but much more rarely — by *Coxiella burneti* and *Chlamydia psittaci*.

2. Other respiratory diseases

M. pneumoniae also causes febrile bronchitis, and sometimes tracheitis. Upper respiratory infection such as pharyngitis, coryza and otitis media are less severe but probably more common manifestations of infection than lower respiratory disease: most are not diagnosed in the laboratory.

Non-respiratory diseases

1. Muco-cutaneous eruptions

M. pneumoniae also causes various types of rash — erythematous, maculopapular or vesicular. In a proportion of cases this is associated with conjunctival and mouth ulceration — the Stevens-Johnson syndrome.

2. Neurological
Signs of CNS involvement are not uncommon in *M. pneumoniae* infection. These most often take the form of meningism, aseptic meningitis or meningo-encephalitis but cerebellar syndromes, transverse myelitis and nerve palsies have been reported.

3. Haematological
Haemolytic anaemia sometimes complicates severe *M. pneumoniae* infection. This is probably due to the development of 'cold agglutinins' — a diagnostic feature of the disease (see below).

EPIDEMIOLOGY

M. pneumoniae infections are endemic in the community but approximately every four years there is an extensive epidemic (doubtless reflecting waning herd immunity after the previous outbreak). The last epidemic in Britain was in 1978–79.

Season: *M. pneumoniae* is a winter pathogen.

Age: most patients are children or young adults: infection in the middle-aged or elderly is rare.

DIAGNOSIS

Serology
Three tests are used:
1. *Complement fixation test* for demonstration of rising titre or — more often — stationary high titres (i.e. 256 or over).
2. *Immunofluorescence* to demonstrate specific IgM.
3. *Cold agglutinins*: patients commonly develop a haemagglutinin for human group O erythrocytes which acts at 4°C. This interesting antibody is probably produced as a result of antigenic

sharing between *M. pneumoniae* and an antigen — possibly I — of human erythrocytes.

TREATMENT

Tetracycline, erythromycin in children.

Recommended reading

Benenson A S (ed) 1975 Control of communicable diseases in man, 12th edn. American Public Health Association, Washington

Christie A B 1981 Infectious diseases, 3rd edn. Churchill Livingstone, Edinburgh

Evans A S (ed) 1976 Viral infections of humans. Epidemiology and control. Wiley, London

Grist N R, Bell Eleanor J, Follett E A C, Urquhart G E D 1979 Diagnostic methods in clinical virology, 3rd edn. Blackwell Scientific Publications, Oxford

Index